the
WELL-BUILT
TRIATHLETE

TURNING POTENTIAL INTO PERFORMANCE

MATT DIXON

VELO.
press

Boulder, Colorado

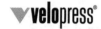

4745 Walnut Street, Unit A
Boulder, Colorado 80301-2587 USA

Distributed in the United States and Canada by Ingram Publisher Services

Library of Congress Cataloging-in-Publication Data
Names: Dixon, Matt, author.
Title: The well-built triathlete: turning potential into performance / Matt Dixon.
Description: Boulder, Colorado: VeloPress, [2014] | Includes index.
Identifiers: LCCN 2014941073 | ISBN 9781937715113 (pbk: alk. paper)
Subjects: Triathlon—Training. | Triathletes.
Classification: GV1060.73 .D55 2014 | DDC 796.42/57
LC record available at https://lccn.loc.gov/2014941073

For information on purchasing VeloPress books, please e-mail velopress@competitorgroup.com
or visit www.velopress.com.

This paper meets the requirements of ANSI/NISO Z39.48-1992 (Permanence of Paper).

Cover design by Pete Garceau
Cover photograph by Nils Nilsen; wetsuit and swim cap courtesy of Roka
Exercise photographs by Nils Nilsen; photograph on page viii by Delly Carr
Interior design by Vicki Hopewell
Illustrations by Josh McKible

Text set in Bembo, DIN, and Melior

19 / 10   9   8   7   6   5

CONTENTS

PART III: TURNING POTENTIAL INTO PERFORMANCE

FOREWORD

There comes a time in every athlete's life when they realize that their methods have to change in order for them to attempt to reach their goals. My "aha" moment came when I plateaued as a struggling age grouper. By the time I was 30 years old, I had toiled away for seven years racing random triathlon events, and my improvement in the sport had been minimal. Why wasn't my effort translating into results?

My story is not unlike that of many other age groupers in triathlon. We put in the time at our "day jobs" to pay for our lifestyle while searching for even more time to stay connected with our family and friends. Add to this the hours of training that we squeeze into every week to fuel our passion for triathlon. I learned to balance all of these important things in my life, and I was making strides in my job and personal relationships. However, my triathlon goals were still far out of reach. I seemed to train more than other triathletes in my situation, yet I was spinning my wheels and not advancing. I was an above-average exerciser but a mediocre triathlete.

Matt has often shared the story of how we met after a cycling class in 2007, noting that I was a wide-eyed, inexperienced triathlete who was "a heavy exerciser." He kindly took a chance on me and invited me to a ride in Marin County to see if I could hang. It was an ugly sight. I am thankful that he saw something he thought he could mold and optimize—gumption. We continue to nurture that quality today because without gumption, our road to success would not have been as vibrant. Even with gumption on our side, Matt had his work cut out for him. He took me under his umbrella and gave this novice age grouper the tools not only to improve but to become a multiple Ironman champion on the journey to world class.

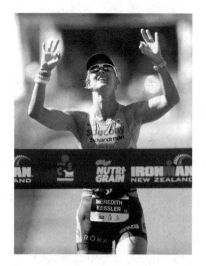

I had one requirement when I began working with Matt and purplepatch in 2007, and it's the same today. I would gladly give myself to purplepatch and his plan for my training as long as he was able to accommodate my busy work and social schedule. I am a firm believer in balance—if something gets out of whack, like excessive training, it can seep into and affect other aspects of your existence. When we started working together, the goal was to turn my chronic exercising into serious, high-quality training. Matt devised a plan that included my 50-plus-hour work week, outings with friends, time with my husband, *and* a power-packed 15 hours of training per week.

Matt's passion and dedication to vastly improving an individual's athleticism can be seen throughout his purplepatch empire. This spirit and vision now radiate throughout the global triathlon community. He has continued to evolve and expand his database of knowledge to the extent that he remains at the forefront of the sport, a beacon for the rapidly expanding triathlon world.

Matching a coach with an athlete is a tricky business. I am fortunate that I found Matt and purplepatch because we are a perfect match. What I know about Matt and the purplepatch philosophy is that *it works*. . . . It works if you want to become a better athlete or triathlete, and it works if you want to find and keep balance in your life.

What I have experienced firsthand and seen with other purplepatch athletes is that Matt will put you in a remarkable position to succeed. From there, it will be up to you. You will be given the opportunity to use his knowledge to achieve your goals in athletics and in life.

It is usually up to us whether we capitalize on special circumstances that come our way. I will always be grateful that I walked up to Matt Dixon and asked for his help in becoming a better, stronger, smarter, more vibrant, and even more balanced triathlete. Do you have gumption? Maybe Matt and purplepatch will change your life forever, too!

MEREDITH KESSLER
6-time Ironman champion
www.meredithkessler.com, www.lifeoftriathlete.com

PREFACE

Over the past few seasons, I have been humbled by the success we have experienced with our purplepatch athletes. Our professional athletes have recorded over 150 victories and podium finishes, including multiple top finishes at world championship events. Not to be outdone by the pros, many of our amateurs have secured multiple wins and world championships in all race distances, and more than 100 athletes have qualified and competed at the Hawaii Ironman World Championship. Despite this success, I don't consider myself a master coach. I am well aware that I still have a tremendous amount to learn. I look around at many other experts in their fields and am humbled by their knowledge and expertise. I am passionate about evolving as a coach, learning from others as well as my own athletes and experiences, and producing more and more top results. So why would I decide to write a book on triathlon performance at this relatively early stage of my career? The answer to this question lies mostly in my own athletic experiences and the reason I began purplepatch fitness in the first place.

My athletic career is a great example of how to "do it wrong." While I managed to take my swimming to an elite level and raced several seasons as a professional triathlete, I do not advise that anyone emulate my approach. Despite my background in exercise physiology and, in the case of my triathlon career, plenty of coaching experience in swimming, I managed to destroy my potential thanks to a recipe made up of massive work ethic, little focus on recovery, and poor nutrition and fueling. I was a world-class trainer, possessing a passion and ability to train that was unsurpassed by any of my training partners, but it only carried me to early retirement and multiple years of very deep fatigue and ill health. I trained myself into the ground and was left unable to exercise at all for almost two years. Ironically, I reflect on that experience with a certain fondness now, as it proved to be the catalyst for me to step back and think more deeply about endurance sports. My athletic experiences, coupled with my education and swim coaching experience, began to frame my set of beliefs about how to properly coach triathlon. These original beliefs remain the guiding principles of my coaching career, and they provide the framework that all purplepatch athletes follow.

By the time we launched purplepatch fitness in 2007, I was already having success coaching athletes of all levels. It may sound egotistical, but I viewed purplepatch as more than simply a coaching business. I was flying back from a race with my wife, Kelli, and she asked what I wanted purplepatch to achieve. My gut response, scribbled on the back of a napkin, was: *To change the way endurance athletes are coached.* Of course as a coach, I want to produce world champions and help my athletes achieve great results! But ultimately, I want to help all enthusiasts and passionate athletes to avoid the common pitfalls, including the one I fell into, and achieve great results in their hobby or profession. In order to succeed at this, I've realized that it is my responsibility to do more than coach athletes—I have to educate, guide, and share ideas to the best of my ability.

This book is simply an extension of the mission I set out to accomplish with purplepatch fitness. It's a guide to what I have learned so far, and it will surely evolve. As I see it, if I don't have more to say in a few years' time, I will have stopped learning, stopped evolving, and therefore stopped improving!

Are You Looking to Improve?

Every athlete sets out with a desire to improve. That personal journey toward excellence may include very lofty goals, such as winning world championships, but I believe that the most important focus is on individual evolution and excellence. As the coach, I view it as my responsibility to lay out the framework, training plan, and supporting elements to help each athlete achieve ongoing success and improvement. I am not interested in trying to achieve quick results with my athletes, leaving a trail of fatigue and destruction in my wake. I am equally uninterested in producing a single world champion if it means my methods destroy others' careers and stand in the way of their improvement. I am proud of many of the results my elite athletes have achieved, but I am most proud of the pattern of success across nearly all of the athletes I have worked with as well as their continued progression and improvements over subsequent years. I firmly believe in the individual and his or her dreams. I take seriously the fact that, while I will continue to have many athletes to coach toward potential success, each athlete only has *one* career and *one* chance. A great coach will never forget that and will do everything possible to help each individual athlete accomplish his or her dreams.

There is great joy in coaching amazing athletes, and I have been lucky to help highly established stars of their sport at the pinnacle of their careers, such as Chris Lieto, Rasmus Henning, and Luke Bell. Wonderful athletes can teach their coaches as much as their coaches can teach them. That said, there is no greater coaching joy than developing athletes from potential into top performance—athletes such Meredith Kessler, Jesse Thomas, Rachel Joyce, and Sarah Piampiano, who began with purplepatch early in their careers, often as amateurs, and evolved to absolute world-class performance. Athlete development, at any level, is the most rewarding aspect of coaching.

So why *purplepatch*? What is a purplepatch? It is where everything falls into place, where you cannot put a foot wrong, and you experience great flow. Of course, we cannot assume that we will be able to live all our lives in the midst of a purplepatch, but we can certainly pursue the knowledge and tools to help make these wonderful phases last longer and become more frequent. This is the heartbeat of our mission.

What You Can Expect

Before we get started, it's important to make a distinction between training and exercising. As athletes, we train in order to pursue a specific goal and to create the conditions for our bodies to prepare for that goal. We train to trigger adaptation in our bodies: to develop the capacity to swim, ride, and run faster in the future than we can now. However, there may be a range of reasons why people exercise: for health, to lose weight, to boost self-esteem or satisfy a healthy ego, or to find community, to name a few. *Exercising*, or working out, is an activity. *Training* is the highly structured pursuit of a goal. As you consider your approach to performance, never lose sight of the fact that you need to train to truly evolve and continuously improve.

I believe this book will help you find long-term success and development as an athlete. The first step is to establish a framework of belief that will guide your decisions around all aspects of training and performance, in the process making you a more confident and successful athlete. From there, I believe that the lessons in this book will arm you with a filter for sifting through the bounty of information that is available through the many channels in our sport.

I hope that this book creates debate. I hope that many smart and informed coaches, athletes, and experts read this book and comment on what they love and hate about the messages inside. Without debate, we cannot learn and grow. I welcome anyone who wishes to challenge my beliefs, but please read with an open mind.

This is some of what I know and understand about performance . . . so far.

MATT DIXON

1

Building a Foundation for Endurance Performance

B ad habits are tough to break, and good habits are equally hard to create. Training endurance is no exception. Many athletes fail to achieve real and long-lasting results because of poor planning, inadequate self-evaluation, and an incorrect mind-set rather than a lack of effort or motivation. Many endurance athletes train hard, but their training doesn't yield consistently positive results. They have access to plenty of feedback to identify the warning signs of faltering progression, but many blindly repeat the same mistakes season after season. It's also easy for athletes to find themselves caught in the weeds, looking for quick-fix easy passages to improvement.

Progress is not achieved simply by wanting it or training harder, and there are no shortcuts. Instead, it takes a fundamental evolution of *mind-set*. If you are not seeing the results you expect, it's time to change the way you look at your sport, your training, and the route you will take to performance. Whether you are beginning your endurance journey or are an experienced athlete who is looking to improve, the first step in your journey is to assess your goals, habits, and training practices and truthfully define your approach to performance. While it sounds like a big project, it is actually pretty simple—and setting your vision and focus before you begin another season of training will reduce the risk of losing your way along the journey.

A ROAD MAP TO PERFORMANCE

Let's begin with one of the most critical components of planning your performance journey. In principle, I could claim that the best strategy is always to head out and train consistently hard, eat well, and ensure that you recover enough to stay healthy. A good performance should be the result. While this approach may seem reasonable, in the real world its tactics and application are significantly more dynamic and complex than they would appear in this summary. Fundamentally, we all have a similar strategy (train hard, eat well, recover, and support our training with strength workouts), but we are individuals with different lives and ability levels. Our history, limitations, and constraints, as well as the way we execute our training strategies in our daily lives, will vary immensely. This brings me to one of the most common problems encountered by endurance athletes of all ability levels: *The ingredients are right, but the cake tastes nasty.*

I believe every athlete understands that in order to improve, there is a need to train hard, train consistently, and train specifically for the demands of your sport. I also believe that every athlete values, at least in principle, the benefits of a solid and healthy approach to nutrition. Furthermore, I believe that most athletes understand the value of high-quality sleep and the consistent integration of recovery into the training plan. Finally, despite some controversy around the "what and how" of implementing it, most athletes believe that some form of functional strength component is a healthy addition to an endurance training program.

Most, if not all, athletes would be quick to agree that these are the components necessary for good performance. Here's their fatal flaw: failing to weave a complete program that values each component equally. When theory is put into practice, athletes place almost all of their focus on the endurance training component, and recovery, nutrition, and functional strength become mere afterthoughts. Before long, life is filled with endurance training sessions crammed into any space that an athlete's life allows, often at the expense of sleep (both quantity and quality), proper fueling and nutrition, and any chance of completing a functional strength session. These athletes train hard, sometimes for many seasons in a row, but fail to achieve real results. They often end up stuck in a cycle of failure. It's not a great route to self-improvement.

So you understand that there is more to finding performance than simply heading out of the door and training—but let's talk about the *secret* of performance. There really is no secret, but there are four magical principles to guide your journey.

Consistency	Improvement will happen only when you apply your training plan in a consistent manner.
Specificity	Your program must be specific to your needs, background, and life.
Progression	Your program should evolve over each phase of training, as well as over each season of training, and even over your entire career of training.
Patience	Real change takes time, so you will need plenty of patience and persistence.

To improve, you will also need to stay healthy, motivated, and injury-free as much as possible throughout your training. Yes, hard work is important, but that hard work needs real support to ensure that you reap the rewards you seek from the effort. By dumbing down your fundamental approach to the point where it is simply training hard, you are setting yourself up for fatigue, burnout, and increased risk of injury.

THE PILLARS OF PERFORMANCE

Your program is no longer about swimming, biking, and running; trying to eat well when you can; grabbing a strength session if you have an open slot; and squeezing in sleep if there is time. You need a *complete approach* that places equal emotional and philosophical value on your endurance training, nutrition, recovery, and functional strength. This simple, yet critical, shift in thinking will give you a foundation for making optimal decisions in training, establish the positive habits that support performance and make them stick, and give you the confidence to maintain a mind-set of "logic over emotion" to review your practices and measure the effectiveness of your hard work. Make the *pillars of performance* the framework of your approach to performance and training. The chapters that follow explore each pillar of performance in more detail, but here's an overview to explain the role of each.

Endurance training. Swimming, biking, and running are the most specific training you do, facilitating the necessary stress to allow sport-specific adaptations and gains.

 Recovery. Sleep and recuperation are required in order for the body to positively respond to that much-needed training load and adapt to become fitter and more powerful. Recovery also includes integrated rest from training and other aspects of your life; specific lighter-stress training sessions; adequate sleep; and specific recovery modalities. All of these combine to maximize adaptation and facilitate performance.

 Nutrition. Simply put, you need to be sure that you provide your body with the nutrients and calories to support your training effort, optimal health, and proper recovery from training. This effort extends beyond healthy eating to include a serious focus on fueling during and immediately after training; the correct quality, quantity, and timing of daily eating; and optimal hydration during, after, and between training sessions.

 Functional strength. Much more than simply a means of injury prevention, a properly designed functional strength program will help you improve your athletic movement patterns; strengthen typically weak muscle groups; and increase your "brain talk," or synchronization of muscle recruitment. This combination will assist in potential improvements in biomechanics, improve your power potential, and likely reduce your risk of injury.

It's natural to be a little defensive about the areas of your training that are underdeveloped, so let's turn to some cases studies that highlight the most typical approaches to training and performance. You might identify with some of these athletes' lifestyle, strengths, and weaknesses. Although I've identified each athlete as male or female, I see the same problems in both men and women.

Case Study | The Aspirational Elite

Johnny is a committed elite competitor who has aspirations of climbing up through the ranks to become a successful professional triathlete. Following a successful previous season as an amateur, he is now in the midst of his first season racing professionally but has recently found himself struggling. Always a very hard worker who aims to train harder than anyone around him, he is now training harder than ever. He experienced grand gains initially, but he is now finding it hard to step up his game. He knows he needs to improve swim, bike, and run to really compete at the elite level, so he is frustrated with his recent lack of progress. It's midseason, and he feels that his power is dropping off. He has also noticed that he is getting sick and held back with minor injuries more frequently, and he has lost a lot of weight in the training process.

Johnny's Self-Assessment

Endurance training. In pursuit of his pro career, Johnny quit his job so he could "go for it." At the end of last season, he dramatically increased his training load (both volume and intensity) to try to make the jump to the next level. Scared of falling behind more-established athletes, he is committed to working his way to the top and fills every day with plenty of challenging workouts. He feels pressure with his early-season races because he was off the pace he had aimed for. He decides to double down on his training efforts to try to catch up in the later stages of the season.

This is a classic case of a strength turning into a weakness. Johnny's motivation and work ethic work against him because a lack of real planning and structure has led to an accumulation of fatigue and a path of failure. Without an extended training history, it is likely that really hard work will create massive gains, as the body is able to adapt. But there will come a time when the constant overload tips the scales, and fatigue and failure are the result. Just how long it takes to reach this point is different for each athlete. The mission is to create a good plan before problems arise.

Recovery. Johnny tries to make sleep a focus and even makes time to take brief naps in the middle of the day, although these are becoming a necessity rather than a recovery strategy. He is not willing to compromise when it comes to his training, so he seldom backs off and integrates a lighter session only if he is truly broken. He reports frequent night sweating, interrupted sleep, and overall fatigue, but his motivation is unbroken.

We are seeing all the symptoms of the accumulation of too much stress. Interrupted sleep, night sweats, and consistent fatigue are big red flags. It seems that training structure is one of the biggest causes of Johnny's fatigue accumulation.

Nutrition. Johnny eats plenty, but he often survives on incomplete meals, such as peanut butter–and–jelly sandwiches, both as a convenience and to save money. He has always believed that lighter is better, so he seldom takes in calories during training and tries to limit calories in the evening to ensure that he drops weight. Johnny hydrates on longer bike rides, but he seldom focuses on hydration outside workouts.

The lack of a real plan for fueling and hydration is largely responsible for fatigue accumulation and failure and often results in athletic starvation. I find it hard to believe Johnny is taking in enough calories, of the right quality and at the right times, to bring about performance adaptations. He is in a state of athletic and nutrient starvation, and the negative consequences will continue if he doesn't make a change.

Functional strength. Johnny started the season with great intentions. He was hitting two or three strength sessions weekly, but this consistency quickly dissolved when his training load escalated. He hasn't thought about strength training for many weeks but has plans to pick it up again in the postseason. This omission is typical and is most commonly a symptom of poor priorities and planning rather than laziness.

This is a classic example of a highly motivated athlete veering off the tracks, headed for a disappointing and short-lived professional career. Every pillar of the self-assessment reveals that Johnny is an athlete without a concise, progressive road map and that he likely lacks the confidence and restraint to stick to a program. Johnny needs to completely reset his approach to training and establish accountability before frustration takes over.

Case Study | The Busy Executive

Mark is a high performer in life, with a great family, a senior position at a finance company, and a passion for triathlon. Since getting the triathlon bug a couple of years ago, he has steadily increased his level of dedication to the sport, despite the demands of his regular life. Not one to fail, and feeling he has a great ability for time management, Mark fits triathlon training into his work life, which includes multiple monthly trips across time zones as well as long, demanding hours. Despite his dedication, his training is often disrupted by sickness, and he is frustrated with his lack of improvement. He often complains that if he only had a few more hours in the day, he could fit in the additional volume and sessions to make those big leaps.

Mark's Self-Assessment

Endurance training. To fit in the training and avoid missing out on too many family activities, Mark wakes up very early every morning to squeeze in his sessions. He hits shorter, more intense sessions in the evenings after his kids go to bed. When he travels, he plans ahead to have access to workout facilities and fits in every key session he can. On his return, he is dedicated to hitting the hard training to make up for a loss of volume. His weekends are made up of early-morning sessions followed by kids' soccer and volleyball and other family activities.

Cramming in endurance training with a volume-centric focus always leads to lower-quality sessions and poor ability to adapt. The result is poor performance. I see this all the time, and I have ongoing battles with executives to try to help them see the logic.

Recovery. The obvious red flag is Mark's very poor sleep. He is often limited to four hours in a night, much of which is broken, and he rarely feels rejuvenated when he wakes up. Generally speaking, he has very little time for rest, and he is accustomed to feeling rushed and manic. He particularly feels the effects of travel, especially when crossing time zones.

Little sleep and the inability to rest lead to a highly compromised immune system, hence Mark's frequent sickness. It is very unlikely that he can make many positive adaptations through his hard work.

Nutrition. Mark strongly believes in a high-quality diet and eats all organic foods, but he often settles for a snack while he works or misses meals altogether. He is frustrated with his waistline, which he tries to attack with a subtle calorie deficit. Mark is convinced that reducing his weight is the key to running faster.

Simply another stressor in his life, nutrition is a problem for Mark. He frequently underfuels and regularly fails to achieve the calories needed to support his training and recovery schedule. His fat retention is more likely due to high stress and athletic starvation, not eating too many calories. If he perpetually exists in an overstressed state, Mark is sure to hold on to that spare tire and fail to positively adapt to training.

Functional strength. Mark doesn't believe strength work has a role in endurance sports, and he has never done it.

Mark would benefit greatly from adding two very short sessions to each week, each one coupled with a swim or run session. These additions should be made in conjunction with a reduction in both the frequency and the volume of his main endurance sessions.

If Mark took the same skills and knowledge he uses in setting up a successful business life and applied them to his triathlon training, he would be more productive. This situation is common among busy professionals and is often related to their inability to stop and review their situation before training. Simply mimicking what other athletes have done in front of them, they fall into a mind-set of "more is better" and form habits that are counterproductive to their goals. Their goal-driven approach to health often comes back to haunt them, with negative effects in daily work performance as well as family relationships. The solution is a smart, pragmatic approach and an athlete who is brave enough to adopt it.

Ironically, Mark's case has many of the hallmarks of an athlete who is frustrated by frequent injuries and ailments. While we likely have a genetic predisposition to be less or more resilient in response to overuse injuries, the frequency and severity of such injuries are undoubtedly influenced by many of our supporting habits and approaches. If you reread Mark's case but replaced the competition for training time with an athlete who is struggling to find training time as a result of being frequently injured, the same lessons are there. In nearly every case I have seen of an athlete with frequent injuries, there is usually a strong influence of improper fueling, underrecovery, and a greater training load than they are able to handle. Just taking half a step back from training, with an increased focus on sleep, fueling, and functional strength, can often radically reduce the time that an athlete spends sidelined by frustrating injuries.

Case Study | Lifestyle Female Athlete

Beth has been competing in triathlons for a couple of years, progressing from a few sprints each year to enjoy the Olympic-distance and even a few half-Ironman-distance races. She loves the lifestyle, challenge, and friendships developed through the sport, and although she doesn't often worry about stepping onto the podium, she does want to improve. Performance aside, Beth also wants to maximize the health benefits of triathlon and gain improved body composition, so she takes her eating, training, and recovery very seriously. However, she has struggled to improve her body composition, and her race times over the past couple of seasons have not improved either, so she is feeling a little frustrated with the sport.

Beth's Self-Assessment

Endurance training. Beth is a creature of habit: She adheres to a very regular schedule of training, seldom missing a session. Much of her training is done at lower intensities with the intention of improving her "fat burning" and aerobic fitness. She finds interval training challenging, and she hates hills during bike and run sessions because she feels that she lacks the power or strength to get over them.

This approach is missing some of the most important elements of successful endurance training. It seems as though Beth does in fact have very limited power, likely resulting from limited interval and strength-based endurance sessions. It's probably the case that Beth rides in an easy, light gear for much of her rides, spinning up hills slowly to make them easier.

Recovery. Beth gets plenty of sleep and doesn't worry about missing a session or two. She doesn't accumulate much fatigue from training and rebounds quickly from any training sessions. She does notice sore muscles following longer bike rides or runs.

Good recovery is the goal, but it is worth looking beyond good sleep and resiliency even when recovery seems to be on track. In this case, Beth might not be stressing her body enough to elicit real change. As a result of a cumulative lack of stress, recovery is not even a factor. It seems her body has simply adapted to her exercise, and she is not training hard enough to elicit real change. Her sore legs following a long and self-reportedly easy ride are a big red flag. This soreness is surely related to issues with fueling.

Nutrition. Keen to improve body composition, Beth tracks almost every meal with diligence. She is hesitant to undo all the "calorie-burning good" her training sessions accomplish, so she rarely takes in calories during exercise. After training sessions, she restocks protein with her favorite meal— a large chicken salad with plenty of veggies. Even with this approach, she just cannot seem to lose the extra fat and is highly frustrated that her hard work is not paying off. Her biggest obstacle to eating well comes in the evenings, when her sweet tooth causes her to crave ice cream or other desserts.

Both male and female athletes are prone to adopt these "healthy" eating habits that will never yield long-term success. When athletes underfuel during and immediately after training sessions, the consequences include massively elevated stress, athletic starvation, and fat retention combined with lean muscle loss. The "athletically starving" athlete will experience poor recovery, loss of power, poor body composition, and a lack of improvements. Beth's nutrition is not supporting her training, and she will never improve without fundamental change.

Functional strength. Beth feels better with strength work and seldom misses her two Pilates classes each week. She doesn't understand how strength work helps her swimming, biking, and running because her power and speed never seem to increase.

There is a significant difference between doing workouts to promote general strength (at the gym or in a Pilates or yoga class), and a functional strength program specifically designed for endurance sports. While regular general strength workouts are a wonderful activity to promote fitness, there is no direct correlation with endurance performance. Beth's Pilates workouts make her healthy, but they fail to provide her with the strength and power work that will lead to improvement in her endurance training.

While Beth spends much of her week committed to training, her approach lacks real planning, progression, and support from her key elements. This is surprisingly common in endurance sports, and many men face a similar set of struggles. The result is that Beth is really simply *exercising* (and staying fit!) rather than actually *training to improve.* With a more complete approach, and with no greater time commitment, she could really see better results.

A SMART, PROGRESSIVE PLAN

These case studies are the stories of real athletes who came to me looking for help. I'm happy to report that in each situation, we were able to make changes that led to significant improvements in performance. If you've had your fill of nasty cake, it's time to change the recipe. Most of us are using all of the right ingredients, but we are not proud of the results. It all comes down to this: You can train your heart out, but without a smart, progressive plan that is supported by equal focus on all of the pillars of performance, you will never realize your best results.

I urge you to take a step back and avoid simply looking at this week of training, or even this month. Instead, aim to establish the habit of effective and smart training. This habit includes consistent hard work, but work that is supported by recovery, nutrition, and functional strength.

PILLARS OF PERFORMANCE SELF-ASSESSMENT QUESTIONNAIRE

To establish your progressive training program, we must first measure each of your performance pillars to determine which are in need of improvement or focus. Your answers to the questions will help you identify specific red flags and sources of increased stress that compromise recovery and adaptation. See Appendix A (page 293) for sample answers.

You are not expected to get a great score, so set aside your ambitious nature long enough to take an honest look at where you stand. The goal is an easy self-assessment of your current approach to your sport. You should be able to answer each question with a simple yes or no. If the answer is sometimes, that's a "no." Some of these questions will raise red flags of poor practice, while others simply showcase a need for a shift in mind-set or approach.

ENDURANCE TRAINING

1.	Is your rating of how your training is going dependent on the number of hours you accumulate in each discipline?	Y N
2.	Do you stick to a regular training template, and are you willing to make changes as you go?	Y N
3.	Do you perform most of your training sessions at a relatively similar intensity?	Y N
4.	Do you plan for rest and recovery?	Y N
5.	Do you follow a classic periodization build of 3 weeks of hard work followed by 1 week of easy work throughout the season?	Y N
6.	Do you place the same emphasis on your swimming training as you do on cycling and running training?	Y N

NUTRITION
Daily Nutrition

1.	Do you often limit your caloric intake or try to hit a particular number of calories with your daily diet?	Y N
2.	Do you avoid fat in your daily meals and snacks?	Y N
3.	Do you rely on carbohydrates as a main or primary source of calories in most of your meals?	Y N

4.	Do you frequently skip breakfast or have a hard time consuming calories early in the day?	Y N
5.	Do you often go more than 4 hours in the day without consuming any calories?	Y N
6.	Are you able to regulate body composition and energy levels without counting calories or putting yourself on a strict "diet"?	Y N

Fueling

These questions focus on the calories that you might consume during and immediately
(0 to 90 minutes) after exercise.

1.	Do you take in calories during any training session that lasts more than 60 minutes?	Y N
2.	Do you always consume calories within 60 minutes of training?	Y N
3.	Do you consume protein within 15 to 20 minutes after most training sessions?	Y N
4.	Do you fear taking in calories during or immediately after exercise due to issues with your weight or body composition?	Y N
5.	Do you focus on hydrating throughout every session, regardless of temperature or intensity?	Y N
6.	Following a heavy training session, do you often get strong cravings for carbohydrates later in the day?	Y N
7.	Do you retain body fat or struggle to maintain proper body composition despite a heavy training load?	Y N

Hydration

1.	Do you consume at least 1 ounce of fluid per pound of body weight on a daily basis?	Y N
2.	Do you consume sugar-based beverages (Gatorade, Monster, Coke, etc.) outside exercise?	Y N
3.	During training, do you hydrate with a low-carbohydrate sports drink (under 4 percent solution)?	Y N

Continued on next page

Continued from previous page

FUNCTIONAL STRENGTH

1.	Do you follow any strength and conditioning program as part of your triathlon training?	Y N
2.	Does your functional strength plan evolve in focus throughout the season?	Y N
3.	Does your strength training focus on group-based classes such as Pilates, yoga, or TRX?	Y N
4.	Do you focus on specific personal weaknesses (mobility, strength, coordination) in your functional strength training?	Y N

RECOVERY

Do you experience any of these symptoms?

		NEVER	SELDOM	SOMETIMES	ALWAYS
1.	Night sweats	O	O	O	O
2.	Unusually sore muscles	O	O	O	O
3.	Fatigue during the day, insomnia at night	O	O	O	O
4.	Fluctuating motivation or depression	O	O	O	O
5.	Changes in appetite (loss of appetite)	O	O	O	O
6.	Frequent sickness (colds, sniffles, cough)	O	O	O	O
7.	Inability to get over sickness (takes longer to bounce back)	O	O	O	O
8.	No performance gains despite training	O	O	O	O
9.	Reliance on caffeine or stimulants to perform at work, in daily life, or in training	O	O	O	O
10.	Frequent overuse injuries (muscle tears, shin splints, sore ligaments, etc.)	O	O	O	O

part I

PILLARS OF PERFORMANCE

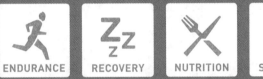

ENDURANCE RECOVERY NUTRITION STRENGTH

2

Stress & Endurance Training

Stress. It's one of those words that you likely hear or say almost daily. It's usually loaded with negative connotations and reserved for the aspects of life that are filled with duress. But if we consider the *role of stress* in endurance training and performance, the word takes on an entirely different meaning. In particular, stress plays a pivotal role in creating positive adaptation. Pressure still exists because stress can either support or destroy an otherwise sensible training approach.

Stress is your best friend when it comes to pursuing your athletic goals, but it can also easily become your worst enemy. Although we need stress to bring about adaptation, we need to pay very close attention to how much of it, and what kind, we bring into our lives.

This chapter is designed to help you reengineer your interaction with your training. I will clarify the role of stress in facilitating endurance performance, explore what types of stress you need to consider in training and life, and explain how stress can dictate your evolution or improvements. Along the way, I will propose a notion that may seem heretical to some of you, but it will forever change the way you think about and interact with your training.

THE EPIDEMIC OF UNDERPERFORMING

Too many highly motivated athletes in our sport never achieve the kind of results they seek from their very hard work. Many of our sport's most committed athletes train long and hard and dedicate an enormous amount of energy to the pursuit of improved race performance. They become extremely, savagely, heroically fit, but they rarely see racing performance improve. *They are fit, not fast.* Triathlon has created an army of fit, tough, committed, focused athletes. But if we look beneath the surface, we are likely to find corrosive levels of fatigue and elevated injury rates. Sometimes the athlete who appears to embody all that is healthy is actually *unhealthy*—on the verge of a systemic or metabolic breakdown. It's all too common for triathletes to find themselves stuck in a vortex of dysfunctional training, believing that the pursuit of success requires an ever-increasing commitment of time and energy. Why does this happen so frequently?

Triathlon is a sport that attracts very committed individuals who are typically high performers in other areas of their life. Part of the problem is the culture itself: Dedicated (dare I say obsessed) athletes are central to the fabric of triathlon. It's a sport that presents several unique challenges, comprising three individual sports blended to make one event. The challenge of training for three disciplines instead of one is easily apparent, and it is an instant catalyst for many of triathlon's most subtle and pervasive problems. Thus, given the character of the athletes drawn to the sport and the sport's unique structure, it's tempting to dismiss what I call problems as inevitable—but there's more to the story.

Unfortunately, it is not simply the nature of the sport itself that leaves so many participants underperforming—in training, racing, and life—relative to their commitment level and goals. Often the way that the athletes approach their training program delivers an accumulation of too much overall stress and too many overall stressors. In turn, the training generates chronically elevated levels of fatigue and stagnant or declining performance.

If your goal is to win the Hawaii Ironman World Championship, everyone would agree that you will need to do a very high amount of training. With this in mind, if I was to ask last year's champions if, despite their wins, they wished they had managed to get in even more training, I am sure that they would look at me as if I were crazy. They know that they did precisely enough training to win—no more, no less. They may recognize an element of luck in the mix, but none would consider his or her preparation insufficient. But more to the point of this chapter, *they did not overdo it.* Had they done so, they would not have performed so well. They did the amount of training their bodies could handle and no more. This is a lesson that triathletes struggle to internalize. Instead, we fixate on the staggering training volume that most world champion professional triathletes endure and conclude that we should train as much as they do in order to optimize our performance. Of course many of us are not aiming to win the overall championship in Kona, but nearly all of us are looking to improve.

The success of your training plan should not be judged by the number of hours you have accumulated. Rather, it should be judged by the level of adaptation that your hours of training have delivered.

OPTIMIZING STRESS AND ADAPTATION

For those of us who have dedicated our lives to the pursuit of performance, it's fortunate that the human body is an adaptation machine. We can be fairly confident that given appropriate physiological and psychological stimulus over time, we will get fitter, stronger, and faster. Unfortunately, adaptation is not a simple switch that we can just turn on. What's more, adaptation can work against us just as easily as it can work for us. Stress creates the conditions for adaptation. The right amount of stress (more accurately, the right balance of stress and recovery) will yield a state of positive adaptation. Too much stress relative to recovery, and the body will still adapt, but it will do so in ways that are undesirable, suboptimal, and in extreme cases nonfunctional or destructive.

What Is Training Stress?

Training stress is any disturbance, triggered by physical activity, of an athlete's overall metabolic and physiological state.

Your training is the necessary stress that should elicit positive physiological adaptations to make you stronger, fitter, and more powerful. If your training approach is appropriate, the stress of training will facilitate positive change. If your training approach is not appropriate, then negative changes (or unwanted adaptations) can occur.

As a training athlete, your goal should be to maximize specific stress while staying in a positive state of adaptation. This sounds simple enough, and it could guide you to make sound decisions throughout your training process. But it's all too easy for highly motivated athletes to lose a sense of logic and fall prey to emotional and fear-based decisions when assessing their training needs. Too often endurance athletes fall into the trap of judging training success by how many hours they can accumulate in a week, regardless of whether their training is actually providing positive change. Let's give this a further twist and think about it from the opposite side: As an endurance athlete, you should do the absolute minimum training necessary to achieve your goals.

I know it sounds radical to suggest that you do the least amount of training possible to achieve your goals, but we've established that it is not the actual amount of training stress that counts. Rather, *it is the relationship between stress and recovery that matters.* This statement is not exclusive to training: Put this way, you can see why understanding all of the stress in your life is so important. As an athlete, you can and should differentiate between two distinct stressors:

Training Stress	Specific, applied, intentional stressors that are critical to facilitate improved performance in your sport
Nontraining Stress	Variable, unpredictable, uncontrolled stressors that you are forced to deal with on a daily basis but are not specific to improved performance in your sport

It is the aim of the professional athlete to minimize variables associated with nontraining stress in order to optimize adaptation for every unit of training stress applied. A professional usually seeks to limit or eliminate "normal" work schedules, prioritize sleep, and keep life as simple as possible. When it is not possible to reduce stress during time not spent training (for example, contract negotiations, holidays with family, or travel), pro athletes typically anticipate the situation by modifying their training load. It is easy for an amateur athlete to understand that great success demands hard work, but they may not appreciate the additional focus that is necessary aside from training. Watch a committed professional athlete spend hours simply lying around the house between training sessions, and the notion of hard work takes on an entirely different meaning! This essential recuperation is mentally challenging and full of its own sacrifices, including loss of the normal social activities that most of us treat as facts of life.

Although many amateurs are highly motivated and have great passion for their sport, most would agree that the goal is to maximize sporting performance within the restrictions imposed by the need to maintain a balanced and successful life. After all, if you win your local Olympic-distance triathlon but get fired from your job, or your spouse leaves you, or your house is repossessed, it would be hard to argue that the win represents real "success." By necessity, your outlook as an amateur is a little more nuanced. Thus, for most of us, success can be more broadly defined as improving in the sport, performing at work, thriving socially, and nurturing positive relationships (with spouse, partner, children, or friends). With this outlook, the goal of the amateur triathlete should be to maximize training load as one part of a vibrant, passionate, and engaged life. I refer to the full picture of your life inside and outside sport as your *global stress environment*. The amount of training you undertake needs to fit within the constraints of that environment in order for you to be successful.

Quantifying Stress

Your training causes hormonal, cardiovascular, and musculoskeletal stress. The trick is to apply enough training stress to create positive change but not so much that you accumulate too much fatigue or get injured. So how do you go about this?

When considering training load, we have to consider the accumulation of stress that our "bucket of life" provides us. I like to call this an athlete's *global stress load*. As you set up your training approach, it is critical that you not only quantify your training stress as one part of your global stress load but also develop an awareness of the various sources of *nontraining stress*.

Nontraining stress arises from an accumulation of all the stress in daily life. This can be a laundry list of stressors associated with work, family, relationships, environment, travel, finances, and so on. Figure 2.1 captures some of the most common sources of stress. These stressors don't provide much (if any) musculoskeletal or cardiovascular stress, but they certainly accumulate and inflict a great deal of hormonal stress on your body. This is an incredibly important point, so let's take a moment to explore it in more detail.

FIGURE 2.1 | SOURCES OF NONTRAINING STRESS

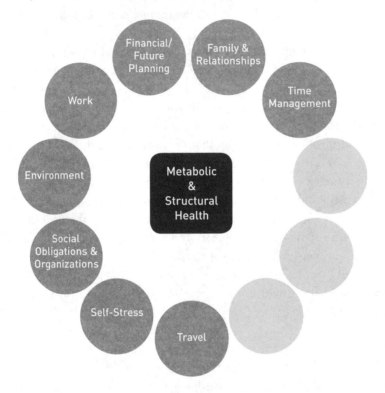

Metabolic and structural health are affected by sources of both nontraining stress and training stress.

First, the endocrine system is massively, mind-bendingly complicated. As much as sport science has taught us about hormones, and as much as we are beginning to understand how hormones regulate everything in our body— including our response to stress—we really don't know all that much. Rather than try to cover what thousands of research papers have failed to explain, I'll focus here on the salient points.

First, simplistically, there are two main hormones we can think about when it comes to stress response: testosterone (T) and cortisol (C). These two hormones work in tandem to create the "fight-or-flight" response to stress. Again simplistically, elevated testosterone is associated with "fight," and elevated cortisol is associated with "flight." But both are triggered by any stress event; what matters is the T:C ratio rather than absolute levels. A stable ratio indicates a high capacity for stress absorption and adaption. Elevated testosterone is better than elevated cortisol, but it has its own problems. This is one of the reasons that hormone replacement therapy is so effective for masters athletes: It resets the T:C ratio back to where it was when the athlete was young, resilient, and capable of handling an enormous training load.

The challenge is that no individual athlete has the resources to track and monitor dynamic hormone levels on a daily basis. This is why it is so important to develop a recovery awareness relative to your global stress load and to understand what life events can disturb these hormone ratios.

You might not associate the stress of a job interview or a poor night's sleep tending to a baby with that of performing hard hill-running repetitions, but all three events create a massive amount of hormonal stress and strain on the system. Although our bodies are incredibly smart, they don't do a great job of differentiating the different sources of stress that suppress our hormonal systems. For the endocrine system, a fight with your boss might have the same effect as toughing it out through a really hard interval session. This understanding reveals the importance of acknowledging the accumulation of stress that we all face in our daily lives. It should also lead you to the realization that the application of training stress needs to be carefully thought out in terms of overall training load and in conjunction with your global stress environment.

Pillars to Support (or Destroy) Adaptation

There is a way to improve your overall metabolic health and offset a lot of the negative stress provided by the accumulation of life stress as well as stress provided by training. Recovery (sleep, rest, and recovery) and nutrition (nutrition, hydration, and fueling) can be your most consistent performance enablers. Of course, recovery and nutrition are no panacea—as is the case with stress and adaptation, the very same things that can lead to stress reduction, mitigation, and balance can quickly become the most destructive negative stressors that you have to cope with. In order to get these right, you must calibrate timing and quantity, and, given the unpredictable nature of life and training, it must be an ongoing effort. Ignore them and you will experience negative consequences—maybe not today, and maybe not tomorrow, but eventually, insufficient recovery or poor nutrition will lead to a state I call "chronic nonfunctional adaptation," which is often referred to as "overtraining."

FIGURE 2.2 | **COMPLETE WHEEL OF STRESSORS**

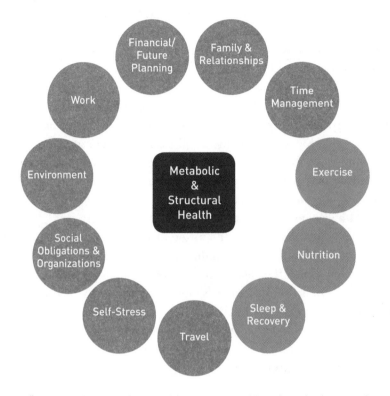

When your "bucket of life" is overflowing with stressors, positive adaptation becomes impossible to achieve because metabolic and structural health are compromised.

When we consider training integration, specifically as it relates to recovery and nutrition, we can complete the whole picture: the "wheel of stressors" that should be considered in setting up our training life (Figure 2.2).

Uncovering Your Potential for Positive Adaptation

Before you dive into planning a detailed integration of your training schedule and the other parts of your life, you should consider another important element of stress and training: Every athlete (and person) responds differently to stress. How you will respond to the stress of an interview or the pressure of endless nights of limited sleep is highly individual. Over time you might even find that you respond differently to identical stress events at different times. It's possible for different athletes to respond identically to similar stress events or to respond differently to identical stress events.

In other words, an athlete's stress response varies over time and depending on the circumstances.

This is important because as humans, we tend to look for patterns in our lives and to ascribe results accordingly. If a given series of training sessions is highly productive, we are inclined to think that the same series will be equally productive every time we apply it. Unfortunately, this isn't the case. Our response to stress impulses will always be shaped by our global stress environment. And, as we all know, our global stress environment is in constant flux.

Exactly the same kinds of variations affect how you will respond to training load and type, which is why it is so important to avoid the temptation of following the training regimen of a professional triathlete. I work with many athletes who are highly resilient—they can handle enormous amounts of training before succumbing to fatigue or signs of nonadaptation. I also work with athletes with similar life stressors and race results who are much less resilient under a similar training load. These athletes are more fragile—they can still have every chance for success, but they must be coached very differently.

A great example of this type of situation is two very different athletes who experienced similar success under my guidance. Linsey Corbin (whom I no longer coach) and Meredith Kessler are both multiple Ironman champions and have raced head to head many times. A few years ago they both toed the line at Ironman Coeur d'Alene, doing battle throughout the race and finishing in first and second place with only a couple of minutes between them. They were both a long way ahead of the rest of their competition.

Although it was a lovely day for both them and purplepatch, the point is that the journey of training they took to get there could not have been more different. At the time, Meredith had transitioned from full-time work into the life of a full-time pro and had years of endurance-based training behind her. She was highly resilient and was embracing the newfound time she had on her hands. She was responding very well to a high-load training plan, with only periodic small bursts of recovery needed to keep her fresh. She was doing a lot more than she had previously and was maintaining positive adaptations.

In contrast, Linsey was coming off a high-load training approach that had left her with various ailments and fatigue. Her situation was very different, as she had a greater tendency to accumulate fatigue and get niggling aches and pains. For her to be successful at this time (she has since evolved back to being able to complete a greater training load), she needed to integrate much more recuperation and recovery into her training. Her focus was on consistency and avoiding too much fatigue. She was completing fewer hours with more recovery and also with more focus on intensity in key sessions.

If I had flipped their plans, their results would have been below par or might even have resulted in injury. This type of difference in approach is worth considering in your own preparation.

Integrate Training and Other Parts of Your Life

No matter your level or experience, in order to set up a successful training program that delivers ongoing success over an extended period, you must think beyond the training that you do. And if you have a clear picture of your bucket of life, you can successfully integrate training into the mix.

Of course, life stressors don't go away, so your mission is to avoid simply dumping a training plan on *top* of everything else in your life. Instead you should aim to integrate the two and maintain an overall state of positive adaptation. *If* you can achieve this, you will be able to create *consistency*, one of the key components of performance evolution.

There is a wonderful story about Abebe Bikila, the great marathoner who ushered in the modern era of Africa-dominated distance running at the 1960 Olympic Games. Bikila won the marathon in Rome, running barefoot, a total unknown. He then virtually disappeared from international competition, running in and winning just a handful of races over the subsequent years, only to return four years later to win again in Tokyo. At the press conference following the medal ceremony, a journalist asked what sort of training regimen Bikila followed, wondering how he had been able to maintain such a high level of performance without racing. Bikila replied that he did not train. The disbelieving journalist probed deeper to discover that after the coup that had ripped Ethiopia apart, Bikila had lost his privileged job in the military and begun working in a coffee plantation in the mountains near the town of his birth. He lived in a village in the lowland, so he would run the distance between the plantation and his home twice a day, in the morning and at night. Upon learning this, the journalist accused Bikila of misleading the world's assembled media, saying that he trained every day, probably running more miles than any other runner in the world. Bikila gently reminded him that this was not "training"; rather, it was simply running as God intended.

In this heart-warming story lie two truths. First, high-altitude training works. Second, Bikila stumbled upon conditions that fostered the adaptation necessary to run great distances, steadily and in difficult conditions. The fact that he also ran fast—after all, he wanted to be away from his family for as short a time as possible—was only icing on the cake.

In summary, at least with regard to integrating an awareness of one's bucket-of-life stress into one's training plan, the key word is "flexibility." You must always keep your training plan flexible so that you can adapt to your global stress environment in a dynamic fashion. If you stick too rigidly to a plan, you risk nonfunctional adaptation. But if your regimen is too loose, you will lose the benefits of consistent application of training stress. This balance, though challenging and requiring constant self-awareness, is mission-critical for the amateur athlete.

DEVELOP A NEW VIEW OF TRAINING STRESS

As you navigate your way through your training life, it is important to understand how training stress will yield results and symptoms that will help you make smart decisions to allow recovery, consistency, and performance improvements. We should embrace the word "stress" as it relates to training because it is needed to force positive adaptations. We disrupt homeostasis in a specific way, and the body should be able to respond and adapt to the stress to make it fitter, stronger, and faster. I will be diving into details of plan creation in Part III, but let's take a moment here to explore how we can and should view training stress.

During workouts and in the hours that follow, you are likely to experience *acute fatigue*. Although it's perfectly normal, I would even venture to say that acute fatigue is a necessary part of training. Feeling tired during or after a workout does not mean you should pull the plug on that session or schedule multiple days of recovery. This is *anticipated stress*. We expect to feel fatigue during and after a session.

That said, appropriate training should not result in massive trauma that leaves you very sore and with debilitating fatigue. Any time a single session leaves you with extremely sore muscles, very tight muscles (holding in spasm), or the inability to recuperate and train the following day, that session was likely too intense relative to your current fitness or level of accumulated fatigue. I call this outcome *unanticipated acute fatigue*, and it is a sign that the session's stress was too great for your body to effectively respond in a positive manner—especially because the required recovery time will be significantly longer. Of course, fatigue is always a tough element to balance, and only wisdom and experience, as well as a little smart planning, can truly enable predictable outcomes.

When you string together multiple days or weeks of training, you are likely to experience an element of accumulated fatigue. This, again, is absolutely normal but is worthy of some consideration so that you can tell the good from the bad. Let's say you head away to a training camp and embark on multiple days in a row of extended workouts, with more workouts in a day than is typical. You will almost certainly accumulate fatigue, but the key is that this is *anticipated accumulated fatigue*. It is a part of the plan and does not call for any action. In fact, it is likely important and highly beneficial to push on with this fatigue accumulation, as you are using the multiple sessions and days to deliver a large training stress. Assuming that recovery will occur soon, this anticipated fatigue can yield very positive results. One of the primary reasons why positive adaptation is possible in this scenario is because at a training camp, you are likely to enjoy minimal nontraining stress.

This is very different than *unanticipated accumulation of fatigue*, in which you experience a slow buildup of residual fatigue to the point that the body falls into a state of nonadaptation. When this occurs, it doesn't mean you are "overtrained," a term that is thrown around far too loosely in endurance circles, but it does mean that ongoing application of training stress *will not yield positive results*. In other words, if you choose to carry on training hard when in this state, you will be unable to adapt to the training stress.

It is critical that you understand and monitor this type of unanticipated stress and fatigue accumulation. When you reach a nonadaptive state, it is an impossible situation because it is the point where injury, illness, or longer-term fatigue is right around the corner. A smart athlete is able to train up to this line, then intuitively respond to the need to back off and recuperate. Once time is allowed for restoration and positive adaptation, it's possible to push hard again. Unfortunately, most of us are not intuitive when it comes to the warning signs of unanticipated accumulation of fatigue, which are described in Table 2.1.

TABLE 2.1 | **SIGNS & SYMPTOMS OF EXCESSIVE ACCUMULATED FATIGUE**

SLEEP	Broken sleep patterns most nights
	Waking up with night sweats in the middle of the night
	Feeling very tired during the day (especially in the afternoon) but wide awake during the middle of the night
PERFORMANCE	High perceived effort with suppressed power, pace, and heart rate relative to expectations
	Inconsistent or poor training or race performance despite good fitness
	Inability to reach higher-intensity speed or power intervals despite good fitness
	Inability to recover from single workouts
	A string of poor results despite seemingly good preparation
BODY AND APPETITE	Unusually sore or tender muscles
	Drastic changes in body composition (inability to lose fat or sudden weight gain or loss)
	Frequent sickness such as colds, sore throats, and fevers
	Inability to get healthy following sickness
	Changes in appetite (can be either a loss or a great increase of appetite)
	Blood values red flags: declining iron, low vitamin D, blood-profile disruptions
MIND-SET	Declining ambition or motivation to train
	Lack of enjoyment or fulfillment in training
	Feeling of sorrow or depression
	Apathy about goals or upcoming races

If you ever experience many of these symptoms, you are likely in a state of nonadaptation, and you must allow rest and recuperation. This condition is obviously a warning sign that your training approach has flaws, but in my experience these flaws are not limited to the number of hours you are actually training. Poor or inadequate sleep, recovery, nutrition, fueling, and hydration all contribute to an accumulation of too much stress. Compounding this accumulation is a training program that is likely too stressful when combined with your bucket-of-life stress.

Don't expect to get through your training year without falling into this state once or twice. It is the awareness of the situation and the actions that you take when it does start to take hold that will allow you to forge through without massive disruption or other negative consequences.

NEW GOALS FOR ENDURANCE TRAINING

What does all this really mean in your training life? I promised that I would suggest an approach to training that might change your perspective on it for the rest of you life. Here it is.

Your goal for your training program should be to achieve great consistency of specific and effective training by minimizing life stressors and maximizing your training load while remaining in a state that allows for steady, positive adaptation. If your life stressors accumulate to the point where they become an overwhelming force in your life, you will have to recalibrate your training load in order to remain consistent and healthy.

Put another way (and very simplistically): *You should be training the least amount possible to achieve your goals.*

I cannot tell you how many times I have been asked by athletes, other coaches, or journalists about the number of hours of training necessary to perform well in triathlons. "How many hours do I need to train for an Ironman?" "How many hours a week do your professionals train?" "If I can squeeze in more hours of training, should I?" All of these "how much" or "how many" questions are the wrong things to be asking and, in my mind, are irrelevant to setting up a smart program.

To be honest, I rarely consider total training hours as a barometer for success; in fact, I seldom even add up how many hours a week my athletes actually train. Instead, I engineer the key sessions that I feel need to occur, then surround them with other supporting sessions that help recovery or preparation or work on another element of endurance performance. The framework of the week is built around two linked concepts: *What needs to get done? When can the athlete accomplish it?*

Once the framework of the training week is mapped, I also need to consider (especially for busy amateurs) if there is time in the week to allow recuperation and downtime. Rather than compressing workouts into every possible window of time in the day, we treat sleep, recovery, and rejuvenation as a part of the program, as much as swimming, cycling, and running. This level of *recovery intentionality* forces the athletes I coach to look at recovery in the same way that they look at training: something that must be accomplished in order for them to consider their training plans successfully executed. If they don't execute the assigned recovery, they have failed. Brutal but simple. (In Chapter 3, I investigate the symptoms of accumulated stress, how to balance fatigue, and tools you can use to ensure that you make smart training and life decisions on an ongoing basis.)

A Very purplepatch Story: Sami Inkinen

One of my coached athletes who provides many lessons for busy working professionals, parents, and aspiring athletes is Sami Inkinen. I met Sami when he was in the midst of launching his tech company (www.trulia.com). He was a classic budding entrepreneur but also a keen triathlete. He had a few years of triathlon under his belt, with some solid results, but had strong ambitions to truly evolve his performance. Unfortunately, these ambitions coincided with all the challenges, stress, and time constraints of building a successful company.

The good news is that Sami, the ultimate pragmatist, is extremely diligent in tracking his sleep, fuel, nutrition, and other metrics in his pursuit of learning and success. We knew that Sami would have restricted hours to train in any given week and that training stress would need to be balanced with the demands of his business. Rather than beginning with the classic question "How much training can you do?," we decided to approach the challenge by first thinking about areas in which we were not willing to compromise. The list included high-quality sleep, proper nutrition, appropriate fueling, and specific key training sessions that could be executed well.

By framing these areas first, we naturally arrived at an allotment of training hours that Sami would typically be able to manage—10 to 12 per week, not a lot for an aspiring elite amateur triathlete. My task was to set up the type of progression and sessions that would maximize the time Sami *did* have. Aside from the occasional opportunity to hit a small training camp or weekend away, we never broke the 12-hour rule, and in many weeks the training hours were even reduced to maintain his health, energy, and consistency. His role was to apply the plan intelligently, and he was charged with making logical decisions rather than emotional ones. Case in point: If he had a board meeting and a trip to New York in a given week, he could not also aim for 12 hours of training. Instead, he would cut intensity and duration in order to retain energy and health. We would delay key sessions to the following week.

What was one part plan, one part crazy experiment led to Sami being one of the most successful amateur triathletes in the sport, with multiple overall Ironman and Ironman 70.3 wins, overall championships at Alcatraz and Wildflower, an Ironman 70.3 amateur world championship, and a sub-nine-hour time in the Hawaii Ironman. All of this took place as he also grew his company and took Trulia public in 2012.

It is obvious that Sami has a great natural ability in the sport and a wonderful baseline fitness and physiology for endurance sports, but his success certainly would not have happened if we had tried to squeeze 13, 15, or 17 hours of training into each week. He would have been fit and fatigued and almost certainly would have failed. Rather than falling into the trap of looking over the fence at his competition and judging his readiness by their training approach, he simply did *all he could to prepare within the constraints of his life*, then raced with an open mind and a willingness to give it a shot. Of course, if he were racing as a pro or not working, he would have been able to accumulate more hours, but his success arrived out of the willingness to be practical and logical.

While we don't all have Sami's engine, we certainly have the capacity to take a truly smart and logical approach to our training and sport.

If you spend lots of time adding up weekly training hours and monthly totals, it's time to put your pen down. If your lens on training success is built around a simple accumulation of hours, you cannot be maximizing your performance potential. While training volume is important, it is a derivative of a sensible training plan, not the objective. Training volume as *the* metric of projected success is nearly immaterial. There. I said it. I am officially, publicly, irretrievably a heretic.

TRAINING ZONES

By understanding the goal of the training session, you can monitor your effort and ensure that you nail the desired result every time.

The Five Zones

ZONE	TARGET	RPE/FEELING	DESCRIPTION
1	RECOVERY	<4 Very easy	Blood is moving, but without big effort.
2	EASY ENDURANCE	3–5 Conversational	You can sustain your effort for extended periods without fatigue.
3	MEDIUM ENDURANCE	4–7 Strong, not breathless	Effort is strong, but you can sustain it for extended periods. Most people would run a half-marathon or half-Ironman in this range.
4	THRESHOLD	7–9 Hard	Maximal steady-state effort, not comfortable. You can sustain effort for several minutes (up to an hour for elite athletes).
5	POWER & SPEED	8–10 Very hard	This is an effort or speed you can hold for just a few seconds up to a minute. It includes all high-end speed work.

You won't find power zones, pace zones, or heart rate zones in this book because I want you to first value and embrace what the feeling and perceived effort should be in each of the zones. Develop a strong feeling of effort in your training sessions, and support that feedback with the metrics and data from tools such as power meters, GPS watches, and heart rate monitors. These tools often cause us to forget how to feel and think. Make it your goal to effectively implement your training zones in a more balanced way.

Defining precise zones in terms of power, heart rate, or pace is helpful if you are looking to create a common language between coach and athlete. You can undergo testing in a lab, a review of your training, or benchmark sessions to arrive at your objective power, pace, and heart rate zones. In working with my athletes, I tend to utilize benchmark assessments most often, but don't overemphasize data derived from one day and one session.

3

Recovery

I find myself talking about recovery so much that I have been called "the recovery coach." I take it as a compliment to be considered an authority on a proven modality of training, though my athletes would smirk at this notion considering the tough workouts I prescribe. I push my athletes to focus on the value of recovery in their training progression and overall plan because it is a catalyst to great performance jumps.

When athletes approach me for coaching services, I begin by asking how they have gone about improving performance in the past. Their answer inevitably involves the number of hours or miles of training, what types of intervals they enjoy, or how these intervals progress. It's clear that the bulk of their emotional capacity is spent designing the swimming, biking, and running portions of their training approach. If I follow up with questions about recovery, nutrition, or functional strength, the common response is "Oh, yes, those too, of course." Although these athletes invariably say that each of these supporting elements is critical to performance, if I review their daily approach to training, it's easy to see that recovery, nutrition, and functional strength quickly diminish to "nice-to-have" status. Over the course of the season, they fall away altogether for the sake of fitting in more training, and recovery is the first casualty.

Most endurance athletes understand on an intellectual level that recovery is essential for training consistency, physiological adaptations, injury prevention, and emotional stability. Nonetheless, many fail to embrace recovery as a part of their plan. I believe this omission arises from a lack of confidence in the approach and plan. As athletes, we tend to gain much of our confidence from those tough workouts and training blocks, but little confidence is gained from resting and relaxing. Coaches have long understood that all of the adaptations that result from training occur during rest. Yet I see coaches fall into the same trap as they map plans for their athletes, relegating recovery to an afterthought. Triathlon coaches are particularly prone to this mistake because we are forced to squeeze not just one but three disciplines into the training plan. Once you shift your approach to training and embrace recovery as one of your four pillars of performance, suddenly the quantity and quality of your sleep is as important as those tough biking or running intervals. Just to be clear, I'm not championing recovery as a shortcut to performance; it is an essential component that will allow you to work harder, more consistently, and with better results. When you begin to see and feel the benefits of recovery, you will have increased confidence in the usefulness of easy sessions or recovery days. A smart training program will never yield optimal results if it isn't supported by adequate recovery (as well as proper nutrition and fueling).

BENEFITS AND GOALS OF RECOVERY

Beyond the obvious strain on muscle and other tissues, training for endurance sports affects your immune system, hormonal balance, and metabolic state. All this hard work stems from a simple desire to improve our capacity to perform in races, life, or both. Triathlon attracts such motivated and committed individuals that I seldom spend time persuading them to train more or train harder. In fact, many triathletes are extremely fit but chronically tired. When I see so many hard, dedicated training hours failing to result in breakthrough performances, I often conclude that an emphasis on recovery will be key to such a breakthrough. Properly integrated into a training plan, recovery will

- Restore the immune system and hormonal balance
- Repair the muscles damaged during training

- Maintain emotional balance over training blocks, seasons, and even careers
- Deliver optimal results from key specific training sessions for better race-day preparation

This chapter details the methods and tools that assist in recovery and regeneration, but first I want to explore the impact that recovery will have on your training and performance.

Consistency: Where the Evolution of Performance Starts

The outcomes of recovery—a strong immune system, muscle repair, emotional balance, and a good yield from key training sessions—all lead us toward the gateway to performance evolution: consistency. *The goal of properly integrated recovery is to open the door to tremendous and lasting consistency of specific, high-value training.*

Consistency is incredibly difficult to accomplish over many training blocks, a season, and even years. So many things can get in the way, including injuries, life events, emotional fatigue, or loss of motivation. I have seen many very talented athletes never evolve toward their potential simply because they were unable to string together any real ongoing consistency.

The promise of creating consistency should have massive appeal for those who buy in to the value of properly integrated recovery. If you are resistant to such words as "rest," "recovery," and "rejuvenation," take solace in the fact that recovery doesn't mean less training! The goal is not to cut back on training, or to attempt to get great results from less training, but to establish a sustainable training load that is specific and elicits positive gains. It sounds quite pragmatic, doesn't it?

When an athlete is able to find his or her own optimal training recipe, there will be a progressive training load over the season, finished off with highly specific fine-tuning for key events. Through it all, there will be a supporting element of lighter sessions, days, or mini-blocks of rejuvenation.

Underpinning all of this is the fact that physiological adaptations and improvements happen during recovery. So even if you are a lover of really hard work, you need to take some easy time to open the door of opportunity to maximize those tough sessions. If you fail to recover, your hard work will become less and less appealing as layers of fatigue begin to creep up on you.

Ultimately, hard work without recovery causes your physiological growth and your motivation to flatline.

If you are always emotionally spent or fatigued or fighting illness, it's unlikely that you are having any fun. This situation will eventually compound until you won't have the mental, emotional, or physical capacity to train hard. When you are no longer enjoying any aspect of the sport, why continue? It will be our mission to integrate enough recovery to support your hard work and ensure that your training progression works optimally. I want you to have a long, enjoyable career of pursuing your goals and pushing your boundaries in endurance sports. It will require hard work over many weeks, months, and possibly years to achieve your big goals; you need a balanced, effective training program that allows you to remain healthy and injury-free so you can consistently complete training that is specific to your training needs. Integrated recovery is the key to unlocking passion, consistent training, and steady progression in performance.

Self-Assessment: Becoming an Active Participant

Many athletes train in an information vacuum without taking into account how they actually feel. They are simply obsessed with the actual training sessions they complete. This vacuum is a very dangerous place. In my experience, athletes who simplify their approach to just training hard, with no other considerations, are less successful. They are prone to peaks and valleys of energy, frequent injuries, or fluctuating motivation—consistency eludes them.

I always tell my athletes that in order to effectively integrate recovery into your training, you have to be an *active participant* in your own training program. Too often workouts are completed simply because they are written on a piece of paper, without regard for your own state of energy, readiness, or accumulated fatigue. It is written, so it must be done. While I don't discount the value of occasionally pushing through a workout, to follow your workouts without listening to the feedback your body is giving you is a mistake.

As I explained in Chapter 2, every athlete handles training and life stresses differently, and every athlete has different life circumstances and constraints. There are common principles and strategies that ring true for all of us, but the specific tactics and practices that an athlete applies for optimal results will vary from one person and situation to another. I want to arm you with as many tools and tactics as possible to optimize your chances of success. One schedule does not fit all, and there is not a one-size-fits-all approach to integrating recovery into your training plan. To be successful, you must become more aware of your daily state of fatigue and readiness. With that heightened awareness, it's much easier to make decisions regarding recovery.

Over the long term, the most effective athletes develop an innate awareness and the ability to accurately predict how they will respond to different types of training and rest. My colleague and good friend Gerry Rodrigues refers to this ability as "athletic IQ." Gerry is talking about more than wisdom or experience; he means the ability, developed through long-term dedication to being an active participant in the training process, to assess and make decisions regarding your approach to training and racing as well as becoming aware of how and why your body feels the way it does. Athletic IQ is something all of us can develop, from the newbie to the pro triathlete. When my professional athletes develop their athletic IQ, it allows me to push them more, build their confidence, and chart a path for greater success—in some cases surpassing what they ever believed possible.

RETHINKING THE PATH TO PERFORMANCE

How can I help athletes make smart decisions and achieve consistent and effective training? I have to sharpen their *focus*—develop their ability to know when to turn it on and when to turn it off. To do this, we have to unwind some of our thinking around performance.

Tough, gritty performances that lead to glory are celebrated in endurance sports. Sayings such as "No guts, no glory" and "No pain, no gain" that espouse toughness and sacrifice often drive our training. Many coaches claim that the only route to high-level performance is daily hard work, which diminishes recovery by making it seem a sign of weakness. Although there is a need for toughness, you also need to be smart and know when it is time to rest. Even a world-class athlete can't turn it on in every single session, every single day. It is physiologically and psychologically impossible to perform at such a high level and to achieve lasting improved performance. Training becomes a matter of survival. The biggest mistake I see athletes make in application of a plan is going too hard on easier days or sessions. This stunts recuperation and limits performance in those tough sessions. We fail to recognize the courage a great athlete or coach must summon in order to pull back from hard work.

Smart recovery is incredibly difficult to execute, but even gladiators rested. At purplepatch we have a saying for athletes who fight hard and never recover: *Be strong like bull, smart like tractor.*

The training that is supported by recovery needs to be challenging. By properly integrating recovery into your plan, you will be able to offset the bigger load of the key sessions and establish a balance of consistent work that is effective. You should realize that your training load recipe requires artistic application and thought and evolves in relation to the dynamic nature of training and life. Ultimately, a rigid approach to training is foolish because it doesn't allow you to react to how your body responds to the stress and load of training. I often tell an athlete, *Let your body, not your expectations, be your guide.* This is not a license to be lazy but an avenue to build success and consistency.

YOUR PLAN FOR RECOVERY

When considering recovery and its role in performance, it is worthwhile to identify the different types of recovery and how they interact. It is easy to jump to conclusions about what recovery should look like for you, but that concoction of remedies might stop short of giving you every possible advantage. Furthermore, the demands of recovery are dynamic, impacted by the changing training load as well as nutrition and fueling (as we will discuss in Chapter 4). We'll take a look at recovery as part of a healthy lifestyle and in support of training, and explore some modalities that promote recovery. While recovery is not a simple mathematical equation, there are ways to quantify how fit and fresh you are or, if you are definitively not recovering well, there are ways to troubleshoot. With a good sense of the recovery landscape and plenty of self-awareness, you can maximize training and retain the best possible health profile.

Lifestyle Recovery

How you lead your daily life will have a great impact on your recovery. Cheat in these areas, and you will absolutely see the impact on your training.

Sleep

Quite simply, sleep is the most important and critical piece of recovery. Along with fueling, sleep is the factor in performance that most endurance athletes ignore. Your body needs high-quality sleep and plenty of it. After all, sleep is when the majority of recovery occurs.

I won't get into the minutiae of sleep patterns and sleep science; let me just point out that the optimal situation is to consistently get eight or more hours of sleep per night. Obviously, this is challenging for many; it if is not possible, then aim for at least seven hours per night on a regular basis.

If you value recovery as an integrated part of training, and if you recognize sleep as the most critical part of recovery, then you cannot continually or chronically minimize sleep in order to fit in more training. You may need to get up earlier than you'd like in order to allow time for high-quality training sessions, but cutting back on sleep (allowing just three to five hours per night) so that you can cram everything in is not a sustainable practice. If you consistently minimize sleep, you simply will not get the desired returns on your training over the long term. You might eke out gains in short bursts, but long-term negative effects will occur. In summary, sleep is the number-one thing you can do for recovery.

If you suffer from lack of sleep, try to optimize your sleep two or three times a week with an additional one to two hours, or sleep for up to eight to nine uninterrupted hours. Begin to notice how the additional sleep results in an increase in energy and productivity on those days. Maximize the benefits you can get from the most restorative phase of life.

 If you are fatigued during the day but lie alert in bed at night, it is a red flag for an accumulation of too much stress and too little rejuvenation.

Naps and Meditation

If only we could all be so lucky, eh? I understand that finding time may be a challenge, but there are big benefits to be had from napping. It's important to recognize that naps are not about making enough time to fall into deep sleep. The goal is to facilitate "power naps," short breaks of 10 to 25 minutes during which you can calm down, relax, close your eyes, and possibly doze off. Brief naps, even for periods as short as 6 to 10 minutes, can restore wakefulness and promote alertness and learning.

In general, I don't advise long naps (60 to 90 minutes or longer) because they can disrupt nighttime sleep patterns, which are a priority. In fact, I want you to avoid entering a normal sleep cycle during a nap because if you don't sleep long enough to complete the cycle, you will wake up feeling very tired and groggy.

If you are unable to doze off, you might meditate instead. Meditation has recently become more widely adopted as a useful tool for enhancing performance and recovery. Though this is not my area of expertise, many elite performers in business and sport participate in some form of meditation.

 TIP *If you get that terrible, groggy feeling after a nap, it's a sign that you are napping too long.*

Training Recovery

It is no surprise that we need to ensure that we integrate enough recuperation into a training plan to optimize adaptations, prevent injury, facilitate consistency, and prepare us for race-readiness. I encourage you to think about how you can more fully integrate sport-specific recovery into your training week, your training plan, and your season—and quite possibly future seasons. Consider how you can use the following practices to train hard consistently for many, many months. For those training sessions that are specifically designed to be lower intensity, the physical stress or challenge will be low. That opens the door of opportunity for an emotional focus on skills, technique, and the more technical aspects of the sport.

Proper Fueling

It's worth emphasizing that proper fueling gives the body a head start at recovering from the metabolic and hormonal stresses of training. To achieve the best results, you must nail your fueling window. Please refer to Chapter 4 for in-depth information on nutrition, fueling, and hydration.

Light Activity

More often than not, your recovery sessions will consist of light activity or, as many coaches refer to it, active recovery. Lighter-intensity, shorter sessions play an important role in recovery. The goal is not to build fitness, power, speed, or endurance; rather, it is to "move blood" around the body to enable recovery processes to occur and to maximize rejuvenation. Keep recovery sessions under 1 hour; closer to 40 minutes would be best.

These sessions maintain neuromuscular firing and prevent athletes from feeling "flat" or tired following days of complete inactivity. It's common for athletes to go too hard during recovery sessions, trying to turn them into "quality" training sessions. Hard work has its place, and I want to make sure you are ready to give those hard efforts when they are called for. If you have accumulated too much fatigue by cheating on your light sessions, you won't be able to give what is needed. Have confidence in your training, and enjoy your recovery sessions when you can.

 TIP *The pace for recovery sessions should be conversational. It's OK to put in a few very fast but very short bits of work to fire the neuromuscular system.*

Complete Rest Days

Sometimes it is necessary to take a day away from the sport, even if only for a mental or an emotional break. Avoid filling these rest days with other duties or stressful activities, or you'll find that your day away from training is not restorative. One drawback to a complete rest day is that athletes often feel a little flat or fatigued on the following day, which can negatively impact their performance. For this reason, you should avoid taking a complete rest day prior to a key training session. We want to maximize performance during key sessions. If you do need complete rest the day before a key session, be sure to extend the warm-up period of that key session.

Recovery Blocks

Consecutive days of rest or of lighter activity allow restoration and rejuvenation following a buildup of higher-effort days. This arrangement is known as a "recovery block," and it is traditionally incorporated into a training program once every 4 weeks—with 3 weeks of building efforts followed by 1 week of lighter work. However, in my experience, an athlete undergoing 3 weeks of continuous building efforts will tend to accumulate too much fatigue over the long term. Most of my athletes practice 10 to 14 days of building efforts followed by 2 to 5 days of lighter activity. Thus, their recovery blocks are more frequent but shorter. This cycle seems more conducive to reaching our goal of long-term consistency and health. By being an active participant in your training, you can test and find what works best for you. Some athletes are more resilient and can handle more work with less recovery. This variation does not make one athlete superior to another; it only means that different recovery recipes are required.

Extended Breaks

I strongly recommend taking 10 days to 3 weeks away from structured training once or twice a year to get a bird's-eye view of your journey as an endurance athlete, particularly for those who train year-round. Step back and allow yourself to rest. It's fine to remain active, but avoid structured training! Be your own guide to find what is right for you. The goal is rejuvenation so that you can resume training refreshed and motivated. It's rare for an athlete who excludes extended breaks to be successful season after season. On the heels of skipped breaks, performances tend to suffer. In the worst cases, complete burnout or chronic injury drives athletes away from the sport entirely.

 If you have a multiyear vision for the athlete you want to become, extended breaks are a critical component to enable consistency season after season.

Triathlon-Specific Recovery

Many triathletes change up their proportion of training per sport during different times of the year. Typically, they use the post-season or early-season months to increase the load of swimming while reducing running and, to a degree, cycling. Running is a sport that places much higher stress on the musculoskeletal system than biking or swimming does. By doing more swim training in the post- and pre-season, you will allow the tissue that absorbs the most strain during running to recover while continuing to work toward your fitness goals. If there is a specific weakness in your swim, bike, or run, then the training mix might look different for you. The post-season and pre-season are ideal for focusing on your weaknesses, improving technique, and laying the foundation of endurance for the challenge of upcoming training.

Within each discipline, the post-season is a good time to mix things up with a little cross-training. You might mountain bike or do cyclocross in the fall and winter, or you might snowshoe or cross-country ski. It's a time for progressing toward your goal by working on fitness, but all the while making space for recovery and rejuvenation to cope with the sport-specific fatigue that accumulates over the course of a season.

Qualitative Recovery Modalities

There are countless gadgets, therapies, and practices that claim to promote recovery. I like to think of these techniques and tools as the supporting cast for global recovery and sport-specific recovery. The right modality, used in the right way, can facilitate recovery, particularly from acute sessions. However, your time and attention should be first spent on outlining an effective training plan, getting consistent rest and sleep, and implementing proper nutrition and fueling around your training.

Although recovery modalities may be of lesser importance, it's worthwhile to consider including some of them as components of your recovery program. Should you find something that works, don't lose focus. In other words, daily habits are superior to all of the recovery tools that cost money! I think that is a good thing.

Compression

Many athletes consider compression clothing to have a positive influence on recovery. For triathlon, this primarily means tights and calf-guards. I would certainly recommend the use of such items during air travel and following tough workouts. The next level of compression gear includes special equipment designed to create controlled compression, such as the NormaTec system and RecoveryPump. While all of these items are potentially helpful and can be added to your arsenal of recovery weapons, they pale in importance when compared with sleep, proper nutrition and hydration, and an effective training plan.

Heat

For most situations, I prefer heat (sauna and steam) to ice for recovery. The literature on using ice for recovery is inconclusive, and I am not a fan of the tightness that occurs because of it. Although ice is an excellent treatment for acute injury, I do not recommend it as an aid for recovery. If you can't do without your ice bath, don't go too cold—50 to 55 degrees works just fine!

Self-Massage

Specific tools and interventions that focus on fascia and muscular release are a welcome addition to your training habits, but it is critically important to follow proper protocol. When you regularly have soreness, tightness, or the onset of an injury, you should see a qualified physical therapist. Self-help tools such as Trigger Point balls and rollers or foam rollers should not be viewed as methods for treating injury. Instead, I prefer athletes to follow a 7- to 15-minute routine that focuses on the whole body (see "Self-Massage Protocol for Recovery" at the end of the chapter). When athletes focus only on tight or "hot" spots, such treatments can aggravate the site of soreness, and the origin of the problem tends to remain unclear. The goal of implementing regular minisessions is to prevent injury and soreness. Regardless of where the tender spots are, you always go through the total-body routine without lingering too long on any one spot.

Graston Technique or Active Release Techniques (ART) are similar to massage, but they can be very effective as injury prevention. These therapies are more related to injury prevention than to recovery, although the return to full mobility and normal musculoskeletal status is certainly a form of enhanced recovery.

Massage

Though this opinion might be upsetting to some, I am not a fan of massage therapy. Allow me to qualify this remark before you shout at the page in disgust. For an athlete in the middle of a training cycle, deep-tissue massage tends to compromise training quality when applied at the wrong time. Too many athletes squirm and crawl on the massage table while well-meaning therapists dig deeply into the muscle tissue. The truth is that plenty of trauma results from this type of work, and this trauma requires real recovery in order to be truly effective. In the scope of a weekly training schedule, massage therapy tends to be followed by heavy training. This training, completed on top of excessive muscle trauma, often leaves the athlete feeling flat and lethargic. It's my opinion that this type of massage is effective only if full recovery can occur over multiple days after a session.

 If you are a big fan of massage, employ it purely as a recovery tool. Request a smooth and light flushing massage without deep-tissue trauma.

Stretching

Here is another fun topic: Don't bother stretching. At a minimum, don't ever employ static stretching before workouts—and most athletes do not need static stretching after working out. While the jury is out on the specific benefits of static stretching, if any, for normal, healthy athletes, I have personally never seen any benefits from it.

The sport of triathlon does not require a significant range of motion of the muscles or joints, unlike, say, ballet. There is plenty of evidence to show that static stretching before workouts does not reduce injury, assist with preparedness to perform, or assist performance. In fact, some studies show that it might harm performance. In place of stretching, I like athletes to focus on joint mobility (which we will take a closer look at in Chapter 5) and employ dynamic warm-ups before selected training sessions. The only exception is specific stretching activities or exercises designed to address a particular issue or limiter, as determined by a doctor or qualified therapist. The good news is that you can gain time in your life by not stretching.

Quantitative Recovery Modalities

It would be a coach's dream to have a clear and consistent quantitative reading of an athlete's state of recovery and readiness to absorb load. Many are trying, and some are getting closer, but we are not yet to the point where any reading or metric can truly tell us the state of readiness (certainly nothing that is commercially available). I believe that we likely won't ever get to that place as, despite the advent of many smart tools that help us make better-informed decisions about training, some human thought will always need to be involved. That said, tools can be of value if they help you become more objective about your recovery. Some companies have truly started to try and crack the code, such as RestWise (www.restwise.com), which has an app that gathers subjective and objective data from the athlete, then provides a recovery score. It is an interesting approach, and the "learning algorithm" begins to track the athlete's data and state of recovery. You don't necessarily have to purchase an app, but there is an evolving scale in your attempts to quantify your recovery status.

It is important to acknowledge that, like data gathered from power meters or GPS, this is information that should start a conversation. In other words, even if you keep a log, monitor pee strips, or have regular blood work, your training approach and plan should not be driven by these factors. They merely deliver some objective data that should be combined with the picture you create from how you *feel*, what your anticipated state of fatigue is, and what your current goals are. Information is powerful, but it is most powerful when considered in the context of your own wisdom, experience, and subjective feelings and information. Never lose sight of this context.

Training Log

You don't need to spend a lot of money on apps or blood work to start the process of reviewing and tracking your recovery status. At a bare minimum, it is helpful to keep a thorough but simple, training log and fatigue report of your sessions and training. This old-school approach is highly effective because it facilitates a review process for the coach and athlete. As a coach, I have no use for a training log that simply tracks the type and amount of training done with just a comment of two regarding the paces or power achieved in the intervals. This doesn't provide much value if it doesn't track fatigue and any red flags in the training plan. The optimal scenario is to keep a training log that includes the following:

- **Training:** Track both planned or prescribed training and the training completed.
- **Perceived effort:** Use a simple rating of 1 to 10 to measure how hard you found the session. It doesn't matter if it is 6 hours of riding or 10 intervals of 30 seconds max effort with 3 minutes rest—simply rate the effort/cost of the session.
- **Motivation/mood:** Again using a scale of 1 to 10, rate your mood and/or motivation for upcoming training.
- **Fueling and hydration:** It is always good to make comments or add detail to help refine your approach.

These metrics will begin to paint a picture of your execution, energy, and management of a prescribed or planned session. You can also begin to learn how you recover by looking back and seeing if two, three, or four days are required to truly bounce back to full energy following a race, big training block, or illness. The key is to be consistent, honest, and logical with the information you have. Remember, just because you are tired and moody doesn't mean you rush for a nap. If it is anticipated fatigue, it might mean you need to toughen up and push through—rest will be coming soon!

Pee Strips

Urinalysis is a relatively noninvasive method of quantifying your recovery status, hydration status, and signs of impeding sickness. While pee sticks are typically intended for diabetics, they have a practical application for endurance athletes.

By taking a sample first thing in the morning and then before and after training sessions, we can begin to paint a more objective measurement of how you are hydrating and recovering between sessions, which contributes to informed decisions on whether to push through or back off from upcoming training.

Again, it's only information, but it should be a huge influence on what you do and inform you about what is going on in your body.

In urinalysis, the following three primary indicators are relevant for endurance athletes.

First a.m. protein (recovery). If there is protein in your urine at first pee, it indicates that you are not fully recovered from previous sessions. It is worth stepping back and considering why or how you are underrecovered. It is not a reason to stop training, but it is information that should make you stop and review the plan. Note that we are not considering protein in the sample taken after training. Post-workout you should expect to have some protein in the urine, assuming you have been working hard enough!

Specific gravity (hydration). By measuring first pee as well as samples taken before and after workouts, you can determine whether your habits during workouts, as well as during life, enable you to retain or regain optimal hydration status. Remember that you *will* get dehydrated in tough and extended sessions, but our purpose is to regain hydration between sessions. We also want to minimize dehydration throughout key sessions and races in order to offset fatigue, so monitoring status before and after workouts can enable us to see if particular hydration approaches are effective or problematic.

Leukocytes (sickness). Typically, you will not have leukocytes in your urine; if they are displayed in a sample, you may be in the early stages of sickness, as they signify a suppressed immune system. It is a red flag, and one that typically calls for you to back off and recuperate. Of course, I have had athletes who look great, feel wonderful, have no other signals, and have leukocytes show up in a test. In that case, we don't run for bed but make decisions based on what is in front of us, hence continuing to train. In most cases, it is shown to be a false reading, whether because of a faulty strip or contamination. Get the information, then make an informed decision.

Blood Work and Health Measurements

The final area of monitoring for recovery and health status is through regular blood panels. This type of monitoring is often reserved for the most serious athletes, those who have a history of fatigue or health issues, or those who simply love the data! I am not a doctor, and while I can read blood panels, I prefer to surround myself with smart people who are experts in their chosen fields. The key in this type of assessment is that you, as the athlete or coach, find a specialist who meets two main criteria: (1) The doctor or practitioner truly understands the athletic lifestyle and monitors your readings and profile through the lens of an athlete, not simply general health; (2) the doctor has a clear and strong history and code of ethics that fit with yours. For me, this means nothing more than honest appraisal of health status with the goal of improving health and drug-free performance. Your chosen doctor should have the strongest ethics, as the vast majority do!

Blood work can provide useful information about your general physiological tolerance to training and monitor your ability to keep up with the increased red blood cells and consequent micronutrient turnover caused by training. Essential components of recovery are ensuring optimal red-blood-cell and hormone recovery and restoring levels of essential micronutrients. Blood-work monitoring allows us to view the exact levels of these vital components of performance and to ensure that they are optimized. It doesn't matter how well you train if physiological factors are not balanced prior to your race.

One of my trusted resources in health and performance well-being is Dr. Garret Rock, a doctor based in Boulder, Colorado, who specializes in orthopedics, chiropractic, biomechanics, and sports and exercise physiology. Dr. Rock has worked with many of my athletes and aspiring athletes at all levels.

The following case studies from Dr. Rock explore the benefits of monitoring your blood work periodically. These are stories of real athletes. Only a few findings are presented; the diagnoses were arrived at after reviewing additional tests and individual histories. *Note: These case studies should not be used for self-diagnosis without a review of your own lab results by a doctor trained specifically to work with endurance athletes.*

Optimal Red-Blood-Cell Turnover

Red blood cells (RBCs) are among the most important factors in optimizing performance. When RBCs aren't optimally healthy, performance suffers. RBCs deliver oxygen to the tissues of the body and are an important player in getting waste carbon dioxide from tissues to the lungs so that it can be exhaled out of the body. The greater the oxygen delivery to muscles and the greater the rate of carbon dioxide clearance, the greater endurance you have.

RBC turnover increases during exercise. During training, the body demands an increase in RBC production in order to keep up with the increased rate of RBC death. This demand greatly increases the utilization of certain micronutrients that play key roles in RBC production. If intake or absorption of these micronutrients is not balanced with the increased usage, a reduction in RBC numbers and/or oxygen-carrying capacity can occur. The result is a decrease in performance.

Case Study | The Ironman–Fatigued Athlete

An Ironman-distance athlete is feeling excessive fatigue. She says she experiences severe fatigue by the midpoint of the racing season every year. She competes in 10 to 15 races per year.

Blood tests reveal mild microcytic anemia (characterized by low RBC volume), low iron, and low ferritin (stored iron). Her findings are consistent with decreased red-blood-cell production and maturation in addition to low iron levels.

Supplementation of iron is prescribed for two weeks, but this treatment yields only minimal improvements in her numbers when a follow-up test is conducted. Further testing reveals decreased intestinal absorption rates of iron, which leads to a gastrointestinal function panel. The test results in a diagnosis of mild celiac disease, which is causing mild intestinal bleeding (unnoticeable in stool).

Doctor's Note: *This case study presents a situation in which the athlete's body is unable to keep up with the rate of RBC destruction being caused by the combination of training and mild intestinal blood loss. The key is to stop the intestinal bleeding by avoiding the allergenic trigger, which in this case is gluten. We made significant dietary changes to help enhance the athlete's iron absorption. Finally, we focused on the athlete's race schedule, organizing her participation in races in a way that allowed for her full physiological recovery after each event before she returned to a program of intense training and racing. After a few weeks of our interventions, further testing following big efforts revealed much-improved RBC recovery and iron absorption. She was set free to race. In the months that followed, she found a gear she didn't know existed, and positive performance results occurred.*

Tolerance of Training

One of the important aspects we look at through blood monitoring is an athlete's tolerance of training. Although there is no single simple test that is a tell-all for how well training is being tolerated by the body, general indicators are found through testing specific hormones and comparing current red-blood-cell indices with previously established baselines. These comparisons allow coaches to further individualize and optimize an athlete's training.

Case Study | **The Overstressed Busy Professional**

An elite triathlete and runner complains of fatigue. She states that her legs always feel "flat," she doesn't seem to recover as quickly following hard workouts, and she is not sleeping well. In answer to questions, she says that she is training 12 to 15 hours per week, is working 50 to 55 hours per week in a high-stress environment, and has a very busy social life. Blood is drawn weekly over three weeks to ensure the accuracy of hormone indices and compared with results from two sets of tests that were done in the past.

Blood-work findings indicate high cortisol (levels of 32.3, 34.1, and 32.6 in the morning, when the blood is drawn, with a normal range being 6.2 to 19.4).

Although cortisol fluctuates throughout the day and during exercise, her results strongly suggest hyperadrenal function, which is a general indication that there is too much stress (physical, emotional, or a combination) on the adrenal glands. The result is a cascade of physiological processes that can lead to decreased immunity, fatigue, blood-sugar imbalances, muscle breakdown, inflammation, fat retention, thyroid hormone imbalances, and more. Unbalanced cortisol levels can greatly influence performance.

Doctor's Note: *In the case of this athlete, a short break from training; nutritional interventions; and a focus on recovery, life balance, sleep, and time management resulted in a normalization of cortisol levels and her ability to race competitively again.*

Micronutrients

Monitoring micronutrients can be an effective training tool for the endurance athlete, most notably for long- and ultradistance athletes. Training increases the utilization rates of many micronutrients. Sometimes utilization rates exceed intake, which can lead to deficiencies that typically alter physiology. For example, deficiencies in iron, folate, and vitamin B12 will directly influence red-blood-cell turnover and lead to inadequate red-blood-cell production and often anemia. Unrelated to RBCs, deficiencies in magnesium due to training or racing in hot, humid environments can lead to potassium deficiencies, which can put an end to an athlete's race day.

There are many examples of the importance of maintaining optimal micronutrient levels in athletes. Burn rates of micronutrients are influenced by so many factors that it is difficult to know exactly how to prevent these deficiencies. Blood temperature, blood pH, rate of absorption, individual physiology, outside temperature and humidity, diet, and effort are just some of the factors that may affect these rates.

Research suggests that the shotgun approach of overloading the body with all micronutrients through supplementation may not prevent these deficiencies from occurring. Therefore, monitoring the most important micronutrients can help prevent the performance deficits that come from deficiencies. Temporary monitoring of micronutrients can also reveal individual micronutrient utilization tendencies.

Case Study : **The Underfueled Athlete**

A professional triathlete appears for routine monitoring. She has transitioned over the last nine months from the International Triathlon Union (ITU) circuit to the Ironman 70.3 (also known as half-Ironman) and Ironman distances. She has generally been tolerating the training well and does not have complaints. Being new to the higher-volume training for these longer distances, she does not know what to expect.

Blood work reveals low-normal hemoglobin (12.0) and hematocrit (36.2), small platelets (mean platelet volume 6.5), and borderline large red blood cells (mean corpuscular volume 99.7). These findings are consistent with two previous tests, which she was told were normal. Micronutrients are tested as well and reveal a mild functional folate deficiency (within normal ranges, but given the high turnover rate of folate in a female endurance athlete, her levels indicate a deficiency).

Doctor's Note: *The red-blood-cell findings are consistent with a functional folate deficiency. This is not uncommon in female endurance athletes, especially long- and ultradistance athletes. Intervention included significantly increasing the athlete's dietary intake of folate. No supplementation was used in this case because folate can typically be quickly restored by ingesting therapeutic levels via the diet. Follow-up tests were performed each week for three weeks with the following results.*

Follow-up	Folate	Hemoglobin	Hematocrit
1	16.2	12.4	37.7
2	18.8	12.7	38.2
3	>20.0	13.1	40.4

Hemoglobin is the protein used by red blood cells to deliver oxygen to muscles. In terms of performance and general health, these numbers indicate an approximate 8 percent improvement in oxygen-carrying capacity. Although there is no equation to calculate how this improvement affects performance indicators, it is well known that increased oxygen-carrying capacity leads to improved performance.

PHYSIOLOGICAL DIFFERENCES

It is important to remember that each athlete is different and responds to stress in different ways. It is currently impossible to accurately predict an individual's response to different stress situations, but we can begin to learn their general patterns and reactions if we pay close attention to ourselves and other athletes. The only way to learn your own tendencies and reactions is to become an active participant in your own sport and journey. This participation might be logging your own training, taking objective measurements to identify recovery and resilience patterns, or even leaning on the help of a skilled doctor, such as Garret, who can help you navigate through the process.

If you do decide to take advantage of regular blood work, it is best to obtain some baseline health data, established during periods of lighter or moderate training loads. You will then have a benchmark against which to compare new information if and when you gain more data during or after periods of high training load or stress. Remember that this kind of information can be useful, but only if it is related directly to your training and racing approach and habits. Otherwise, it just becomes meaningless data.

Recovery for Older Athletes

I have worked with more stubborn athletes than I can remember—the ones who believe they remain indestructible as they age—and I gain plenty of satisfaction from converting their mind-set and then their performance. The smartest and most successful athletes don't ignore the fact that they are aging; they embrace it as a great platform of fitness and take the chance to hit even more specific training to yield results. Here are some key considerations for aging athletes.

Slower recovery process. In general, the body is slower to adapt and recover from tougher sessions. This means there is less margin of error for retaining a logical mind-set in training approach and more need to embrace the requirement of very light sessions and days in order to achieve great results.

Increased impact of higher intensity. High-intensity training sessions have high value but also a great impact on your body. Older athletes should only hit very high intensity once or twice in each week, with a greater reliance on supporting low-intensity sessions to bridge the hard days.

Loss of strength and mobility. A properly designed strength and conditioning program is absolutely key because muscle integrity is compromised with age. The emphasis should be on retaining and improving joint mobility, but there should also be a focus on strength and power.

Loss of top-end VO$_2$max. As we age, our maximal ability to deliver and utilize oxygen for aerobic exercise decreases, but properly designed training protocols, including some higher-intensity training, will reduce or delay the effect of this reduction. If the athlete simply relies on logging miles or hours at low to moderate intensity, then this capacity declines.

Now for the good news—*we retain endurance as we age!* Our capacity to endure remains with us like a bank account of fitness, so aging athletes do not experience much decline in fitness.

Because we are lucky enough to retain a great deal of our ability to keep going, our goal should be to keep going at as high an output as possible. This means we need to concentrate on areas that tend to assist a higher output, such as strength, mobility, higher-intensity sessions, and speed work. Of course, due to our reduced capacity to recover from the work, strength and high-intensity training need to be supported by plenty of very-low-intensity sessions.

The final word on aging and recovery is: Train a little less and hit some high intensity. But support the high intensity with plenty of very easy work, all the while listening to the signals your body provides.

Recovery & Body Composition Issues

Recovery is not often correlated with an athlete's body composition, yet many athletes train hard, often for many years, with less-than-optimal body composition. The solution is never simple, yet athletes and coaches seldom look beyond calories consumed during and outside training to try to improve body composition. I see many trained athletes, frustrated by their body composition, placing themselves on restrictive nutrition protocols without success. One look at them training, and I can *see* the stress they are carrying. Watch athletes in this situation go through a tough set of intervals and fail to achieve a great effort, or have the will to truly suffer and work, and it is obvious that their eating habits are not the central cause of body composition issues and often only contribute to the root causes—overstress and underrecovery.

One of the more delicate areas of coaching is guiding and managing a female triathlete who, despite heavy training, experiences poor performance and body composition issues. There are obvious sociological and psychological ramifications in many of these cases, but the issues often arise because of a lack of understanding or direction. Many athletes get caught in a cycle of failure with training and body composition, and it truly takes a long-term approach to create radical shifts in behavior and attain great results. It can be done, though.

Case Study | The Athlete Struggling with Body Composition

Sharon is a serious amateur triathlete who has trained consistently for several years, but she struggles with declining power and performance, broken sleep, and retention of body fat despite the training load. She is always careful with her food choices and controls her caloric intake.

This is one of the more common scenarios I see among incoming athletes, and it is important to realize that it is not only a female issue. Many male athletes struggle with similar situations, and it isn't a problem with a single solution. However, over the past few years, I have found that when I have an athlete who is training hard and retaining fat, I need to reduce training and increase caloric intake to improve performance and body composition. "Train less, eat more" has become a mantra for those aiming for real improvement.

I think it is important to review these types of cases through the lens of a coach, not a dietitian or nutritionist. I am seeking performance improvements. In the case of Sharon, there are almost certainly multiple factors at play. These are some of the key areas that I would investigate.

Recovery. Is she truly embracing recovery in her plan, both in terms of making the easier sessions easy enough (in terms of intensity) and embracing the need for sleep and proper recuperation? Typically, frustrated athletes double up on training and chase intensity or big efforts in more and more sessions. The training becomes the fat-loss trigger, so lighter sessions and sleep get compromised in the pursuit of burning more and more calories. The result is an accumulation of stress and fatigue, causing a cascade of performance and stress-related responses.

Fueling. In daily eating, the very first place I would look is the calories taken in during and immediately after training. There are often glaring holes, with the vast majority of athletes grossly underfueling and limiting intake after sessions. The result is underrecovery, a great accumulation of stress for the body to manage, and a high propensity for poor food choices later in the day.

Overall caloric intake and quality. Few athletes take in the required calories to support their training, but athletes in this type of situation are even less likely to fulfill those needs. Underfueling, as mentioned above, will lead to cravings for starchy and sugary carbohydrates that are hard to suppress. Athletes in Sharon's situation often have large swings of heavy restriction offset by guilt-promoting gorging on carbohydrates, and these cycles lead to fat retention and energy swings.

Restriction of macronutrients. All macronutrients—fat, protein, and carbohydrate—are vital to us both as humans and as athletes. Unfortunately, fat and/

or carbohydrates are often seen as "dirty foods" and are frequently reduced in or eliminated from the diet. A complete review of a balanced approach to meal makeup is necessary.

My intervention with Sharon would be based on these points, but it would need to be multidimensional and long-term. Removing the scale, increasing recovery and specificity in training, radically increasing post-training fueling, and replacing starchy carbohydrates with high-quality fats and plants would almost surely be priorities. We would aim for a six-month progression of training, recovery, and proper fueling and eating habits, with success parameters being based on energy and mood as well as life and sports performance. If we nail the good habits, then improved body composition will typically follow.

As you can tell by now, recovery doesn't mean taking a shortcut, and it doesn't mean that you will get more from less. There is no denying that the demands of this sport are great, and to achieve great success, you need to be willing to work hard consistently over many months and years. The key is that recovery is a part of that journey. It is an important element of your plan and approach and should be embraced as one of the keys that can unlock consistently high-value training. We don't take recovery time because we are lazy, and we don't run away from fatigue.

Recovery is not simply taking an occasional day off or making sure we get plenty of sleep. It is a complex and dynamic mind-set and collection of practices that support your training, allow you to maximize your hard work, and facilitate training and racing consistency. It is one of the reasons I feel humble pride when I am tagged as "the recovery coach." Bring it on. That is all I have to say.

SELF-MASSAGE PROTOCOL FOR RECOVERY

This protocol is "prehab," a preventive measure that aims to forestall common aches and pains as well as prevent hot spots from progressing. With this protocol, you are *never* aiming to diagnose or cure injuries. Remember that in the case of many injuries, the place where you feel the symptoms often is not the root cause of the actual problem. Hammering away at a hot spot is unlikely to help or cure the cause and may simply inflame the symptoms. For this reason, *always follow the entire protocol, but do it no more than a few times weekly*. This session requires just 7 to 15 minutes.

FEET		Scan the foot for any areas that are tender. If you don't have a Trigger Point ball, a tennis or lacrosse ball will work fine. Gently massage the foot and hold over the tender spots a little longer, letting the weight of your leg fall into the ball to cause mild release of the tension.
LOWER CALVES, MIDCALF		The foot is plantar flexed, but the calf should remain relaxed so the massage can be more effective. Take care to target the center and the inside and outside of the leg. Use your crossed leg to apply more pressure on the area, and sink deeply into the area of focus—the "belly" of the calf. Maintain relaxed and deep breathing throughout.
ANTERIOR (FRONT) SHINS		Roll the soft tissue on the shin, taking care to not apply pressure directly to the front of the tibia (bone). This often forgotten muscle will thank you for a little attention.
QUADS		Use long rolls both up and down the quad. When you get to the outside portion of the quad, you can shift from side to side, but do not go past midthigh or roll the outside of the knee. We want to avoid the lower IT band, just outside the knee. The pain is typically high here, but it is because this is where the nerve bundles end. Don't mistake normal pain signals for injury. You can do more damage than help in that area, so leave it alone. A tight IT band typically originates from higher up, around the hips and/or lower back.

Continued on next page

Continued from previous page

HAMSTRINGS		Massage the inside and outside portions of the hamstring, followed by more specific hamstring work as needed. Maintain relaxed and deep breathing.
GLUTES & EXTERNAL ROTATORS		Massage the glute max. By crossing your leg over your knee, you can reach the deeper stabilization musculature, but remain relaxed and calm. Shift to the outside of the glute to reach the external rotators, using body weight to allow the muscles to relax.
ADDUCTORS		Roll along the inner thigh. Don't forget to breathe.
LOWER BACK		Cross your arms and roll the lumbar spine. To better reach the lat, extend your arms over your head, but aim to keep everything supple and relaxed. Holding tension won't allow the foam roller to provide the intended massage and release.
MIDBACK		Roll the middle of the back, then shift your body left and right to target the outside of the back. You can remain relaxed and allow your body weight to sink into the foam roller.
SHOULDERS		Support your body weight on the hips and roll the back side of the shoulder, which is often sore in swimmers. This area can be tender, and it is worth noting that shoulder mobility exercises are key. Help this area with a focus on these muscles every time you use the foam roller.

4

Nutrition

By now you are well aware that I rank nutrition as a pillar of performance, meaning it holds the same emotional and philosophical value as the other components of triathlon performance. Here's the truth about nutrition and fueling: Getting them wrong can and will limit performance. Getting them right won't hold you back. Note the distinction. If you nail your daily eating habits, integrate a smart approach to fueling throughout and following training, and support your training with proper hydration, there is no guarantee that your performance will improve. Good nutrition and fueling simply build a platform for more consistent training and help promote a positive yield for your hard work. Eating well won't make you a champion, but eating poorly will surely prevent you from reaching your potential. To this end, *consider your eating habits as part of your training program.*

If I were to ask you about the role of nutrition in endurance performance, I'm sure you would tell me that it is key. Although in theory athletes rank nutrition as highly important, in practice they tend to undervalue it. Nearly every athlete I work with has plenty of room for improvement in their approach to fueling both training and racing when we first begin the process. I'd venture a guess that the same holds true for you.

Don't worry; I am not trying to turn you into a monk. I won't ask you to weigh your food portions, and I won't tell you to stop having that glass of wine or beer (I am English, after all!). I do want you to focus on creating smart, easy eating habits and supporting your hard training efforts with nutritious food.

When it comes to nutrition for an endurance athlete, it's important to realize that there is more to it than daily caloric intake. A successful strategy will clearly address these four components:

Daily Nutrition	Breakfast, lunch, dinner, and snacks. In other words, the eating you do aside from fueling your workouts.
Fueling	The calories you take in during and immediately after training and racing.
Daily Hydration	Hydration throughout daily life, aside from training and racing.
Exercise Hydration	Fluids consumed during training and racing.

Why would we draw such lines in the sand? First, the approach required for each aspect of nutrition is different, so it makes sense to discuss them separately. In addition, treating these areas as separate topics with distinct goals helps athletes clear up much of the confusion that reigns over endurance nutrition and create a framework for successful habits.

It would be disingenuous to offer advice on endurance nutrition without first explaining where I stand on this frontier and the rapidly expanding scientific research that informs it. Endurance nutrition is in an extremely exciting time. We are seeing a great divergence in beliefs in key areas such as hydration, the role of macronutrients (carbohydrate, protein, and fat), and other key areas. Research is being conducted at breakneck speeds, and highly regarded experts fall into wildly different camps of opinion on any given subject. With this, you should realize that I am not a dietitian and have not dedicated many years to research and study on this topic. What I do have to offer is a strong background in exercise physiology, a long history of coaching, and a significant amount of time spent talking with the experts and reading their research. Perhaps my greatest influence and nutrition mentor is Stacy Sims, PhD.

The time and effort I have invested have guided how I work with athletes, and I've seen practical benefits arise out of my experience. That said, it would be

LOW-GLYCOGEN TRAINING: CAN I RESTRICT FUEL TO TAP FAT?

There is plenty of research that seems to indicate that training with low glycogen teaches the body to use more fat. Yes, this does happen, but it's not beneficial to you as an athlete. Here's how it works: You use more fat during exercise, signaling the body to store more fat. Access to greater amounts of fatty acid does *not* lead to improved performance, just unwanted training adaptations and impaired immune function.

To affect body composition, use training and food timing to maximize adaptations—fuel before training, eat real food (not just sugary sports bars and gels) during training, and hydrate well. Fueling for workouts in this way will allow you to hit intensity and/or duration with the least amount of negative stress (i.e., cortisol production). Next, really take advantage of the post-exercise window, both the 30 minutes immediately after your session, in which you should take in some protein to maximize cellular adaptations and reparation, and up to 2 hours afterward, when you should eat a balanced meal consisting of a high-quality protein, a good source of fat, and some higher-quality carbohydrates.

Some interesting research is being conducted on endurance athletes utilizing lower-carbohydrate fuel sources, with increasing dependence on fat for fueling during and after training. However, except for purely anecdotal evidence, the research is too young for definite conclusions to be drawn. I expect that carbohydrate will always be an endurance necessity even if we are able to also draw energy from fat or protein in racing.

foolish for me to drive a stake into the ground regarding any of the key topics that create the most debate, such as hydration and macronutrient roles. What I *can* do is lay out the key elements that my background, experience, and study have helped me define for athletes. This chapter is not about resolving the arguments around the finer details of training or race-day fueling, but I hope it will help you filter information that you hear and read, set clear priorities, and develop habits that support better performance. The debates will continue in the world of endurance nutrition, and the available knowledge will grow, but I believe the fundamental habits that facilitate performance will remain the same.

THE PERILS OF NAVIGATING NUTRITION & FUELING

Most triathletes exist in a state of total confusion on the topic of nutrition and fueling, but it certainly is not due to a lack of information. In fact, we are inundated with so much information that it is barely possible to get through a day without stumbling upon free nutrition advice, the next best diet to follow, or a series of quick tips to find more power through nutrition. We live in a world of fad diets, watching the rise of an empire of supplements and quick-fix solutions while a crowd of expert voices offers conflicting information on the subject of what to eat and drink. Even if we manage to identify reputable resources, we still have a winding path to navigate.

The headlines broadcast that carbohydrates are bad for us, yet we are told in the same breath that carbs are the endurance athlete's essential fuel. While some preach that pure carbohydrates are the way to go on race day, others guide us to add protein. We are told to load up on sodium before and during hot races, but read the research and it seems that cramps are not attributable to sodium loss. We are told to stay hydrated for performance yet heed the warnings about too much hydration. The sheer number of experts and quantity of conflicting research makes for a minefield of information. Various companies and credentialed individuals appeal to athletes with evangelical fervor, promoting their views as the only reasonable path. It strikes me that everyone is talking about slightly different things, but the debate is so heated that as an athlete it's difficult to see the difference.

There is one fundamental aspect of nutrition that athletes and experts fail to recognize: the needs of the athlete around training versus the need to create a platform of daily health. In other words, what you take in during and immediately following exercise plays a very different role (performance and recovery) than what you take in outside training and racing (general health). It is impossible to make smart decisions about the quantity, quality, and timing of calories that you take in if you are mixing your training and racing intake with your daily life choices. As obvious as this may seem, it is a huge issue for many triathletes, especially those worried about body composition or weight. Triathletes fall into the trap of underfueling in their training out of fear that they will end up with excess body fat—after all, it is now commonly accepted that sugary foods are a leading contributor to many of the health issues and obesity that dominate the Western world. This notion is born of confusion and a lack of clarity about the differences between fueling and daily nutrition.

ATHLETIC STARVATION:
BREAKING DOWN THE PHYSIOLOGY

When you train "on empty," or without replenishing calories, you place huge stress on the body.

- Low glycogen (stored carbohydrate) levels impair both exercise intensity and training adaptations through reduced post-exercise signaling actions—in other words, optimal adaptations from the training stress will not be initiated.
- Low glycogen availability reduces glucose availability for the immune and central nervous systems. This increases the risk of infection and chronic fatigue.
- Body composition is adversely affected because athletic starvation increases cortisol, a stress hormone, which leads to increased adiposity, or fat that is stored subcutaneously.

The consequences of underfueling are explored later in this chapter; it is enough to say that this habit is rampant among triathletes, and it contributes to a lack of recovery, increased stress on metabolic health, and the same negative implications for body composition and weight that athletes were trying to avoid from the start. I call this habit "athletic starvation," and most triathletes are completely unaware that it's taking root in their daily lives. The vast majority of my incoming athletes take in *too few* calories to truly support their training load. With athletes who are seeking to improve body composition while continuing to train, I typically have to guide them to *train less and eat more*. What? Surely they will end up heavier than they started! Actually, this seldom occurs.

Athletes who are focused on body composition take delight in training to burn calories. Because they don't want to ruin all that good work done, they skimp on the calories they put back in, especially those nasty sugars that make us fat! And so starts a cycle of high stress, with the athlete burning calories but underfueling during and after the workout. Physiologically, this cycle is best summarized as a process of underfueling, underrecovery, and eventually athletic starvation. The end result is a loss of functional mass (muscle) and a retention of nonfunctional mass (fat), which is good for keeping us alive but bad for riding or running hard up hills. As the negative results take shape, the natural tendency is to perpetuate the cycle: Train more; eat less. And so it continues, with degrading body composition, lack of recovery, loss of power, and accumulating fatigue. This mind-set is fed by the confusion surrounding fueling and nutrition. Almost every case of deep fatigue that I see in athletes has a nutritional component. And I have not yet even touched on the accompanying psychological impact and loss of self-confidence.

The big problem in the performance equation is that many athletes eat the wrong thing at the wrong time, creating poor results relative to their potential. Most athletes are grossly underfueled for their training, yet they overconsume poor food choices in daily life. The result is reduced training effectiveness, compromised body composition, and poor performance. Although nutrition remains a complex and evolving subject, it must be a part of your overall program. I will steer you clear of specific diets or rating different types of energy bars. Instead, I want to focus on a method for fueling that supports your training load and a daily diet that allows you to remain healthy. Get these two things right, and you will rise above the fray.

THE BENEFITS OF GOOD NUTRITION & FUELING

I've stopped short of promising that good nutrition and fueling will add up to good performance, but let's explore the solid foundation that good practices can provide and how it may translate the hard work of training into a strong performance on race day.

Maximizing performance in training & racing. Nearly every training session and race requires the intake of additional calories to maximize performance. The longer the race, the more critical fueling becomes, but good practice must begin in your training sessions. While you may be able to "get through" most training sessions without additional calories, this approach doesn't necessarily set the stage for optimal performance. Additional calories can often enhance performance in a given session. Furthermore, you must look beyond the start and end of any single session. I prefer to view training sessions as rolling into one another to facilitate consistency in both training and performance. In other words, the calories that you are taking in during a morning bike ride may have a positive effect on that session. They might also promote recovery from that session and preparation for the run session you have planned for the evening. The right approach will take into account the entire fabric of the training plan—what you have done recently and what is next.

Promoting recovery. For many with limited training time, promoting recovery is perhaps the most useful benefit. Recover well, and you will be able to train effectively more frequently. Recovery is the yield of the hard training you do. You cannot optimize recovery and adaptations without proper timing, quality, and quantity of fueling calories during and after each training session. Overlooked by many, prioritized by the best, fueling is the elixir of performance.

Limiting overall metabolic stress. Exercise is an enjoyable form of stress relief, and the correct dose is certainly highly beneficial as a health benefit, but much of our training includes higher intensity and longer durations than typical "feel-good" exercise sessions. This additional load creates the critical strain to force physiological adaptations that help us gain endurance, strength, sustainable power, and fitness. It is key to performance, but it comes at a cost. During training, your stress hormone, cortisol, skyrockets in response to the training load. We don't want cortisol to remain high following the session. Proper nutrition during the "fueling window" will help bring stress hormones down quickly and reduce the need for stress management over the rest of the day. Less stress, more energy, and good performance in both training and life are not bad things! Proper fueling allows us to achieve the optimal balance that every athlete should aim for: *adding more stress during the training but then doing everything possible to limit the stress once the session is complete.*

Managing weight & body composition. There is plenty of talk of athletes trying to reach their "race weight," but less is said about true management of both body composition and weight. By optimizing your nutrition approach, you should be able to create positive habits that, in the longer term, will bring about positive changes in both weight and body composition. Unless I am working with a mathematically minded athlete who carries no emotional burden associated with weight or body composition, I try to avoid focusing on metrics or interventions. Crash diets and other drastic weight-loss strategies seldom work because they force the athlete into a very restrictive lifestyle that does not lead to successful habits in the long run. Furthermore, given the amount of training most triathletes do, dieting and other interventions are rarely necessary. Positive habits will nearly always yield positive results because the athlete can gain control in a more healthy, sustainable way. It does take patience because forming better habits requires more time than most interventions allow.

Building a foundation for overall health. You are what you eat, right? In many ways, that saying is true. While we all seek performance gains, and good fueling habits make that possible, your performance evolution relies on a platform of solid health. You need to be healthy to adapt to the training load you place on your body—a simple yet important reality. Proper daily nutrition will promote general health and support your immune system along the way. Eat often, eat plenty, and create a strong platform for health.

FUELING VERSUS NUTRITION

If there is one thing I would like to ingrain in you, it is the ability to differentiate between fueling and nutrition. Whenever I talk with athletes on the grand topic of nutrition, I begin here. I find that distinguishing between the two concepts can remove some of the emotional baggage from fueling during and after training and provide a clear, simple framework for all of the other decisions you need to make about food. Eating the right thing at the right time is key for athletes, even if one of the goals is improved body composition. Focusing on the number of calories consumed might be the correct approach for an overweight, inactive person, but it's a short-sighted strategy for athletes who are actively training. Both the rules around nutrition and the individual's needs are very different.

Fueling

The calories and hydration consumed just before, during, and immediately after exercise constitute fueling. The goals of fueling are to

- Optimize performance during the training session
- Allow proper recovery after the training session (thus setting up the next session)

- Facilitate self-control and high-quality food choices throughout the day by diminishing the cravings that occur as a result of poor fueling
- Limit metabolic stress associated with athletic starvation

The fueling window begins 30 minutes prior to a training session and extends throughout the session and 2 hours beyond the time when it ends.

It's important to have an appreciation for what you are trying to achieve with calories and fluids during the fueling window. The correct mind-set will help you go about the task of fueling with a sense of purpose. *All calories taken in during the fueling window are consumed to support training performance and recovery.*

My definition of fueling is performance-driven, and for good reason. I don't want you to think about fueling as a means of supporting good health. I also don't want you thinking about body composition or weight management during your fueling window. Good health and better body composition begin with proper eating management. Get your fueling right, and you open the door to a cascade of good things both for your sport and for your life in general.

It is important to acknowledge that the best sources and types of fuel are highly individual. I would never endorse a single sports product as the answer to every athlete's fueling needs. That said, here are some general guidelines.

Pre-workout fueling. You need to take in some calories 30 minutes prior to training to help establish fuel reserves for longer endurance sessions. This is perhaps most critical if you are training first thing in the morning because even shorter morning sessions are beneficial for lowering cortisol levels, which are high first thing in the morning. The optimal fuel source will contain some protein with a little carbohydrate and a high-quality fat. In general, you want to avoid anything that spikes your blood glucose immediately prior to training.

Fueling during training. Here the key to effective fueling is little and often. Any session longer than an hour should include fueling both to help promote performance during the session and to lower the deficit and stress created by that session after it is over. Most, and some would say all, of these calories should be from carbohydrate, typically a glucose/sucrose combination. However, extended-duration or low-intensity training can absolutely be supported by "real food" options that include plenty of protein and fat. Your ability to

TABLE 4.1 | FUELING DURING TRAINING

CALORIES	3 to 4 calories per kilogram of body weight per hour (3–4 kcal/kg/hour)
HYDRATION	10 to 12 milliliters per kilogram of body weight per hour (10–12 ml/kg/hour)
FREQUENCY	Every 7 to 20 minutes from the start of training until the end

effectively absorb calories during exercise is greatly diminished because the blood that typically helps absorption is busy shuttling oxygen and other nutrients to the working muscles and cooling the skin. To overcome this diminution, you need to dilute the calories with hydrating fluids and take in smaller quantities of fuel at regular intervals. Use high-quality fluids, not just water, to prevent dehydration and the reduced blood volume that induces fatigue. Choose a very-low-calorie drink with a little sodium added to help absorption. Your caloric intake, combined with effective hydration, will ensure that you achieve the goal of training intensity and caloric-deficit reduction. Table 4.1 details basic guidelines for how much to take in and how often. Keep in mind that there will be some variance among athletes.

 TIP *Sessions under 1 hour do not typically require fueling during the workout, but post-training fueling remains a critical component of overall success.*

Fueling immediately after training. We want to "turn off" the stress of training immediately after the session, and your post-session fueling is a huge help in this. Making protein the primary post-training fuel will stunt the cortisol response of training and help begin the resynthesis of muscle tissue (the recovery process). Within 15 minutes of the end of your session—every single session—you should aim to consume 15 to 20 grams of protein. Combine protein with carbohydrate, as the carbohydrate will be used to replenish your depleted carbohydrate (glycogen) energy stores. Many athletes get these calories from a shake or drink, simultaneously fueling and rehydrating, but if you gain these calories from real food, be sure you also drink plenty of water.

Fueling with a post-workout meal. The immediate intake of calories after training is focused mainly on stunting cortisol and beginning the initial replenishment of glycogen, but the job is not yet complete. Eating a post-workout meal replaces the depleted calories and promotes the recovery process. This meal should come from high-quality real food that includes protein, carbohydrate, and fat. Eating this meal within 90 minutes or so of your training session should prevent hunger cravings later in the day. In the 90 to 120 minutes following your workout, your metabolic rate is still elevated, and your absorption of carbohydrate is higher than it will be for much of the remainder of the day. In addition to a post-workout meal, you will want to continue the effort to restore your hydration status to a normal level, but outside actual training, tap water will suffice.

Nutrition

The calories and hydration consumed during the remainder of the day make up your nutrition—typically breakfast, lunch, dinner, and snacks. The primary purpose of nutrition is to support a healthy life. This is where you gain the building blocks of a high-quality diet: the vitamins, minerals, and other advantages associated with good eating. Your choices around nutrition do not directly affect the performance of a single training session, but good nutrition choices support training by

- Boosting your global health profile—lowering the risk of disease, maintaining a strong immune system, and supporting good energy and sleep patterns
- Replenishing depleted resources from your training, such as vitamins, minerals, and macronutrients
- Contributing to optimal body composition
- Assisting in the recovery process by repairing and strengthening tissue, tendons, and ligaments
- Promoting good daily energy levels

Keep in mind what you are trying to do with the calories and fluids taken in during the nutrition window, and the proper actions are more likely to flow from there. *All calories that you take in should provide a foundation for good health and a strong immune system while also meeting your needs for energy and body composition management.* Great athletes are built on a foundation of good health.

For athletes who need to improve body composition or lose weight in order to improve their performance, the nutrition window is the time during which it is safe to slightly reduce calories. This will work only as part of an effective fueling strategy. Mistakes in fueling lead to the downfall of many hardworking athletes seeking to improve body composition. Poor fueling and the subsequent cravings for subpar food choices during the nutrition window make for a pretty miserable existence. In fact, poor fueling may well be the culprit in the poor relationship that many athletes have with eating in general. At the end of this chapter, you will find some simple guidelines for good nutrition.

HYDRATION

The topic of endurance hydration is one of the most contentious in the field of performance nutrition. This is most likely a result of the massive promotion of sports drinks to the wider population as a whole as well as the dangers of over-consumption of plain water in endurance events and the consequent dilution of electrolyte balance known as hyponatremia. Hyponatremia is a dangerous condition that occurs when the level of sodium in your blood is abnormally low. It generally occurs in endurance athletes when they hydrate with water *only*. Remember that our "body water" is not distilled water—it has electrolytes and glucose in it.

Within the pages of an endurance sports publication, you could read a lot of contradictory messages: Drink only when thirsty, but avoid dehydration at all costs; ensure that fluids contain carbohydrate and electrolytes, but water is the elixir of energy and health. Confused yet? Let's simplify things and attempt to provide a basic framework around your hydration strategy for training and life.

The Performance Effect of Dehydration

It is worth knowing that you will become dehydrated while training and racing. Despite this fact, few experts would claim that chronic dehydration assists endurance performance, but keep in mind that overhydration is a potentially deadly scenario, especially if it includes hyponatremia. It's helpful to understand what happens to your body as you become more and more dehydrated.

Perhaps the most significant impact of dehydration is a reduction in total blood volume. Your body is a closed system of blood circulation—blood is pumped from the heart, circulates around the body, and then returns to the heart (via the lungs) to be pumped once again. This process highlights the three important roles of the blood during endurance exercise:

- Deliver oxygen and other nutrients to the muscles for energy production (and upload carbon dioxide and other agents for removal)
- Assist with absorption of calories that are typically consumed during exercise
- Dissipate (through the skin) the heat that is created by the work of exercise

Of these, dissipation of heat is the most important from a health standpoint. Work, in this case exercise, generates heat, and heat is extremely destructive if we are unable to dissipate it. As we continue to exercise, our plasma volume (which makes up between 50 and 60 percent of total blood volume) is reduced. This leaves us with a lower blood volume, and a competition for blood delivery ensues between muscles and skin. The intestines quickly raise the white flag because caloric absorption is the least critical factor in this battle. As dehydration continues, the competition becomes more fierce, but the critical nature of heat dissipation means the skin will continue to win out, leaving less blood delivery to the muscle. The result is impaired energy production and the perception of fatigue.

Hydration & Thirst

There is ongoing debate about how critical hydration is to performance, but one can assume that it becomes more and more important as the duration of the event increases. Either way, I work under the premise that maintaining blood volume and utilizing fluids to ensure the calories ingested during exercise are adequately diluted for optimal absorption make hydration important in training and racing. This is why I would never prescribe ingesting only water; nor would I recommend consuming a very sugary sports drink in every session. I also don't prescribe to the "more is better" belief in hyperhydration. We have a long-evolved natural brain signal that can potentially help us gauge many of our needs—thirst. While many experts suggest that thirst is the best route to judge fluid intake, it's been my experience that many athletes don't have that level of self-awareness. I encourage you to "listen" to your thirst but suggest that you aim for fluid intake of 10 to 12 ml/kg/hour. In cooler conditions, you can be at the lower end of that spectrum, and in warm or humid conditions, you should be at the higher end.

What you choose to drink during exercise should be similar to the natural chemistry of the fluids in your body. This is the logic behind adding a very slight dilution of carbohydrate and sodium to your bottle to increase the rate of absorption. Throughout the rest of the day, you are eating plenty of foods laden with electrolytes and calories, so simply consume water or your favorite beverage. *Avoid all regular sports drinks and sodas throughout the day.* There is no value to any sports drinks or soda outside the designated fueling window.

With the principles of fueling and nutrition solidified, we can revisit the topic of body composition and weight management. Let's set aside performance for a moment. I see many athletes run into health problems and psychological issues because of their relationship with a combination of training and eating. Too many athletes use training as a weight-loss approach and then dabble in extreme diets to accelerate the benefits. This approach never works in the long term.

If you truly want to improve your body composition while also prioritizing performance, you have to have a positive relationship with the fueling aspect of the sport. Proper fueling can act as the catalyst for minimizing stress, making good food choices later in the day (in proper quantities), and allowing the body to positively adapt to the appropriate training dose. Remember that the nutrition, fueling, and hydration pieces of the puzzle cannot be considered as mutually exclusive entities if you are an athlete. Eating less does not promise weight or fat loss. Long-term gains and improvements can be achieved only with long-term positive habits; with a great training approach, supported by adequate recovery; and with an approach to nutrition that supports both your training and your platform of health. Get the *big picture* dialed in, and you will stop thinking that every energy bar you consume during a four-hour ride is going straight to your hips!

GUIDELINES FOR A SENSIBLE APPROACH TO NUTRITION

Eat a good breakfast. I have never seen a successful eating plan that includes restriction early in the day. This is a good time to take in any starchy carbohydrates you may eat as well as plenty of protein and fat. Breakfast is the bedrock of a day of good eating.

Hydrate for energy. Support your daily energy with the regular intake of hydrating beverages. Avoid sugary sports drinks; instead opt for water, tea, or even coffee.

Eat your fruits & veggies. An essential source of vitamins and minerals, fruits and vegetables should be well represented in every meal. Simply put, I have never seen anyone get fat from eating too many fruits and vegetables.

Embrace the fat. Many of us grew up hearing that fat would make us fat. I sometimes wish that this macronutrient could be given a different name without the negative connotations. Fat is essential to good health, supporting the immune system and overall well-being.

Proteins are your athletic building blocks. Each meal should include a portion of high-quality protein.

Get carbs from fruits & veggies rather than other sources. This is not a rule, but it is a good guideline for the nutrition window. Many of your carbohydrates can come from highly nutritious vegetables and fruits rather than from starchy sources such as bread or pasta.

Warm up in the afternoon. Drink a warm beverage in the middle of the afternoon to help raise your metabolic rate, which naturally dips around that time. You will feel more alert and be less inclined to reach for the low-quality, sugary foods.

Eat often & snack plenty. If you are following the above guidelines, you will need to eat plenty and often to support your training load and maintain energy and caloric balance. Nutritious snacks play a big role, and remember that all snacks should include some protein.

Don't diet. As an athlete, you should never diet to lose weight. Instead, create positive habits that yield long-term results. Athletes who go on crash diets seldom have success over the long term.

Recover at night. The best evening snack will include 15 to 20 grams of protein (for example, a nonfat Greek yogurt) to maximize recovery during sleep. Eat a little snack about 30 minutes prior to bedtime, and sleep like a baby.

Don't count your calories. I have yet to have an athlete succeed with long-term athletic performance and/or weight management by keeping strict account of caloric expenditure or intake. It is a dangerous and distracting game for the training athlete, and the negative emotional attachments to food that arrive with this rigid approach certainly outweigh any positive control gained. Focus on habits, not numbers.

5

Functional Strength

Almost every magazine or website aimed at endurance athletes features strength exercises designed to target the core and other muscle groups and, by extension, improve your performance. Functional strength is another hotly debated topic within training and coaching circles. Many successful triathlon coaches decide not to integrate any strength, mobility, or power work into their training programs beyond what is achieved within swimming, cycling, and running. Other coaches tout strength training as equally important to, or even more valuable than, specific swimming, cycling, and running training. On one hand, from those who dismiss strength work, we hear about the marginal value of traditional bodybuilding or generic strength, Pilates, or yoga programs that have no specific relation to triathlon. On the other hand, disciples of strength work often dismiss the necessity of sport-specific training, claiming that work in a gym can effectively prepare any athlete for triathlon competition. Throw in the buzzwords and fads that inform different perceptions of strength work, and it can be difficult to know whether strength training is the starting point of endurance performance or a complete nonstarter.

It will come as no surprise that I believe functional strength is a critical addition to your overall training program. However, this is not a charge to head off to the gym to lift heavy weights, join a Pilates class once or twice a week, or do hundreds of crunches to get strong abdominal muscles. I define a successful functional strength program as resistance training to target mobility, stability, strength, and power to improve the movements necessary for your specific sport and to uncover optimal performance gains. This chapter provides the background information necessary to understand what functional strength has to offer for endurance performance, explains what a smart functional strength program looks like, and offers guidance to help build a program around your individual needs.

Before you get started, it is critical to recognize that no strength training can be a replacement for any swimming, riding, or running that you do. If we think of training as a dartboard, our sport-specific swim, bike, and run training fits squarely into the bull's-eye, and nothing else hits that close to the center. A properly designed strength program will circle that bull's-eye and allow you to maximize the performance yield from swimming, biking, and running. If your strength program isn't built around your specific needs for your sport, you are effectively playing on two dartboards. There is limited value in getting strong for strength's sake. Strength does not make a great triathlete. How much you can bench press or leg press is mostly irrelevant to endurance performance, so a high-quality program will not have you spending time trying to reach new benchmarks. In the same way, how flexible you are or how many crunches you can perform also have limited impact on your performance. It seems like common sense, but I regularly see triathletes following one-dimensional programs. Your strength plan needs to run parallel to your endurance training and your racing season and be viewed as an ongoing key supporter to your coordination, mobility, strength, power potential, and resilience as an athlete.

WHERE STRENGTH TRAINING GOES WRONG

Most athletes instinctively value the role of strength training within the performance program, but there's a great deal of confusion about how to implement a program that truly helps performance. When I begin working with a new athlete, I ask about his or her approach to strength training. Among those who realize the value, nearly every athlete's approach includes either a weekly group-based class, such as Pilates, yoga, or TRX training, or a regular 20- to 30-minute "core and ab" workout they do on their own. The program seldom has any specific progression and almost never considers the progression of the greater triathlon season. This is the norm, and for those who dismiss the value of strength training, such a program is evidence of its futility. There are two truths here: (1) Nonspecific strength sessions simply won't maximize your performance potential, and (2) repeating *any* program without progression cannot continue to yield results. Such an approach ends up being a waste of time.

Some athletes restrict strength training to a couple of months in the off-season so as not to compete with their endurance training and racing. Others begin each season with dedicated focus on strength, but it fades as the endurance training ramps up and eventually disappears from the weekly regimen. This cycle continues year after year; the start of each season is greeted with promises of a renewed focus on strength, only for it to fade again. In both cases, we can attribute these shortcomings to the fact that triathletes lead busy lives, not to mention the priorities of training, but the lack of progression also plays a significant role. Begin *any* strength program, and you will feel results very quickly, as happens with most eager triathletes during the off-season. Repeat that same routine week after week, and it quickly becomes stale. There is no increased load to force new adaption. Results slow to a halt, and now the time spent in strength training provides no emotional or physical benefit or validation. It's only natural that, as fatigue from regular training builds and racing begins, a boring and stale strength component is no longer a priority.

A minority of triathletes have a year-round progressive program, which yields the results needed to truly provide enhanced potential in swim, bike, and run training.

THE BENEFITS OF STRENGTH TRAINING

It's worth repeating: I don't want you to perform strength work to get stronger for the sake of being stronger. I believe that implementing a specific, progressive strength training program will improve your performance, help you avoid injuries, and ultimately allow you to enjoy the race-day experience more because it will be easier.

Lifting heavy weights, or performing an exercise under a load, requires force production. The force required will be equal to the mass you are lifting multiplied by how quickly you move through the range of motion in the exercise (force = mass × acceleration). As with every form of stress, the body aims to adapt. Here's what it looks like in terms of your physiology:

- Neural recruitment (i.e., how well your brain talks to the working muscles) is improved.
- More muscular fibers are recruited into the usable mix, thereby increasing strength and power potential.
- Muscle fibers morph into more efficient muscle types.
- Tolerance for anaerobic exercise, or sustained higher-intensity exercise, increases.
- A host of other positive metabolic, hormonal, and general physiological changes occur.

All of these adaptations are linked to improved athletic performance. Keep in mind that the body uses only as many muscle fibers as are required to maintain the level of work. When you incorporate specific higher-intensity strength work, your body demands that you recruit more muscle fibers. Once you develop the ability to access these fibers (in other words, get your brain "talking" to the typically dormant fibers), they become part of the usable mix. Such an increase simply adds to the potential of power output, or sustaining output when fatigue occurs. Furthermore, all of these adaptations have a practical application to improving sustained power/speed throughout your swimming, biking, or running as well as improving your resistance to fatigue and overall efficiency. Performance isn't just about going faster; it is also about building a broad platform for potential and maximizing our ability to adapt to the hard work undergone in the specific disciplines. The benefits from a properly designed functional strength program ultimately lead to movement synchronization and coordination, improved biomechanics and form, greater overall athleticism, and heightened injury prevention. Now I have your attention, as these are widely acknowledged to be the fundamentals for endurance performance. A solid strength program truly unlocks your potential to improve as an athlete.

Synchronization and coordination. Watch many triathletes, and you will see plenty of effort, often without real control or awareness. Sometimes how you do something is as important as whether you can do it. Most triathletes can do a lunge, for example, but can they perform the motion smoothly, under control, and in a balanced manner? Your coordination and synchronization can only improve through a specific strength plan, which can translate to potential improvements in biomechanics, efficiency, and power production.

LIFTING WEIGHTS: WILL I BULK UP?

You don't have to bulk up, or significantly increase muscle mass, in order to reap the benefits of strength training. This is the primary concern I hear from endurance athletes. In reality, significant increases in muscle mass occur only when a program is designed specifically for that purpose. Unfortunately, many endurance athletes who are strength training, usually under their own guidance, do much of their work in the very range that causes muscle gain: programs designed around moderate weights, high reps, and several sets. This is why so many athletes avoid strength training altogether or stop their program when they enter racing season. We are not interested in that type of program, and the approach we take will easily avoid most or all muscle-mass gains. The truth is that most endurance athletes really don't need to worry about the bulk factor, as they likely don't have the genetic background to build a whole lot of muscle mass in the first place. In addition, you almost certainly don't have enough excesses of the necessary nutrients (dietary protein) needed to build muscle tissues. However, if you are trying to build muscle, you will still need the proper building blocks—dietary protein, and an excess of it in terms of what you would normally see in an endurance athlete's diet. All this being said, we avoid the risk through the design of the program.

Muscle recruitment. Improved muscle recruitment throughout the entire range of motion of a given movement results in all your muscles working together in balance instead of stronger muscles compensating for weaker muscles. This improvement allows an increased amount of *effort* to go into locomotion. Being stronger, when developed properly, can increase your potential to produce force. More potential force production equals the ability to produce more power—for example, to run faster with less effort. Here's another way to think of it: You should be able to generate a given power output with less effort, meaning you should be able to hold a certain pace for a longer period.

Remaining healthy. We all understand the intrinsic benefits of maintaining good health, but strength training unlocks the holy grail of endurance sports: being able to train consistently over many months without having to take time off for injury recovery.

A well-designed functional strength program will improve the movements of the body for sport-specific benefit. Many triathletes have years of the same forward-motion training (running, biking) or a lifestyle that is weighted heavily (pardon the pun) on sitting at a desk job, hence compromising the body's ability to move well. Interestingly, as children, we all had the ability to perform basic movements rather easily. If I look at my young son, he naturally moves into a deep squat position multiple times daily—it's virtually a resting position. Ask any adult to perform this exercise, and it is impossible for many because our range of movement has deteriorated over the years. Likewise, for many athletes, the proper form is surprisingly difficult.

The first part of any program is developing good form and full range of motion through a movement. We can then progress through adding load, complexity, and specificity. It is more important to use the proper technique and utilize the designated range of motion than it is to get strong in a limited range. This means that your thinking must evolve to *prioritize form over load*. It is valuable to correct some of the imbalances we've accrued and improve the way we move during the process of getting stronger. This highlights the need for a progressive program: Within the context of your season goals, a progressive program will define the appropriate time to focus on mobility, power generation, or maintenance.

THE FUNCTIONAL STRENGTH SEASON

Keeping the big picture in mind will empower you to progress both toward your key events this year and toward your vision of the athlete you want to become. Consequently, I recommend setting up a season of functional strength training as part of a cyclical, multiyear approach that will evolve year after year as necessary throughout an athlete's progression. Start by focusing simply on a single-season progression. It should be laid out, typically, with a focus on improving

- Mobility
- Foundational strength
- Stability, coordination, and synchronized movement
- Power production
- Injury prevention and enhanced recovery

This long-term progression must be balanced with the immediate goal of getting ready to perform your best for your "A" race, which is why the types of exercises and the purpose of each workout will change and evolve as the season unfolds. Functional strength over the course of an endurance season of training and racing can be broken down into three progressive phases. The progression should seamlessly flow from one phase to the next, beginning with a greater number of exercises that focus on only one or two areas, such as upper-body mobility and upper-body strength. As the season and program progress, the focus of the exercises becomes more dynamic, incorporating more areas—so two exercises might combine into a single exercise that focuses on both upper- and lower-body mobility and strength. The final phase includes fewer individual exercises, but they are all total-body exercises. Because weaknesses and mistakes can be less noticeable in the total-body exercises, proper form and execution are critical in the more isolated exercises early in the season, in which weaknesses and mistakes are clearly exposed.

PHASE I ⋮ Foundational Strength & Stability

Increased mobility
Improved motor control and balance
Strength progression in key exercises
Stability development
Heightened movement patterns in the kinetic chain

The starting point of any program is to determine your own individual mobility and strength limiters. You can use the functional strength self-assessment at the end of the chapter (page 99) to do this. Any such areas that prevent proper form should be emphasized in your program. Very basic exercises are the bedrock of this part of the program, including learning how to stand properly, squat (or sit!) well, and connect the chain of muscles in an effective manner. Ironically, this phase of the program is where you may report feeling the greatest strength gains, but what is really happening has more to do with pure muscle recruitment and the development of optimal movement patterns. We are effectively teaching the body how to maximize the tools it already has! Because this part of the program demands isolated focus for so many exercises, there are a greater number of exercises in any given session. Note that, due to the specificity of isolated movements, it can sometimes be a little more difficult to see the connection between these exercises and the movements for swimming, biking, or running. Be patient—we get there, but first we need to work on basic movements and overall athleticism.

Strength training tends to fall into the "something is better than nothing" category, so I tend to encourage athletes to go a little *too easy* rather than too hard. We want to end up in a great place, but a conservative beginning is always great. It's imperative that you set yourself up with proper body movements that translate to good form later in the program.

By the end of this phase, you will have improved posture, better-controlled movements, and increased overall strength in core-competency movements. Early in the phase, the load is minimal, often utilizing no more than body weight, but over the typical 12 weeks or so of the phase, you will reduce repetitions and increase load/weight. In other words, as the phase progresses, the focus shifts to building strength, albeit with all exercises executed with great form.

PHASE II ⋮ Synchronization & Power

Further focus on mobility
Increased stability through more complex movement patterns
Heightened muscle strength and power
Improved neuromuscular control in sport-specific activity

Following the initial phase of strength, which normally coincides with the post-season, as well as part of pre-season endurance training, you should have improved mobility and stability and have experienced some strength gains. Much of the gain in strength has come from establishing correct motor patterns as well as improved neuromuscular recruitment. In other words, there is much strength still to be gained! If you were patient in your progression through Phase I, you have "earned" the ability to increase the complexity of the exercises and to increase load in some. We want movement to progress into real strength, and then strength into power, all without compromising endurance performance or joint mobility—so a careful prescription and session planning are needed. You need to be an active participant in your own training and be aware of your level of fatigue or soreness in your muscles.

As you transition into this phase, you will notice that we begin to reduce the number of key exercises, and the more isolated movements in Phase I are grouped into larger movement patterns and exercises. We still maintain the foundational core, mobility, and stability exercises that require ongoing attention, but the strength-focused exercises transition to more sport-specific, complex movements.

This is where synchronization and power come into play. We want to take the improved control and strength and transfer them to more dynamic and power-based activities. You will quickly see that if you skip the initial phase of the program, you cannot effectively achieve all the gains that are available in Phase II. It is worth noting that this phase is the highest impact and leaves the greatest residual fatigue, so you must consider your endurance training in conjunction with these sessions. You should also anticipate that your legs might lose a little "zap" in training. Early-season races can certainly be affected by including this type of strength work, but it is a worthwhile trade-off for the benefits that arise from the work.

Be prepared for heavy-load strength work early, then a transition from pure strength to power—exercises that ask you to move weight quickly. As you progress, your load might actually go down because you have to add the speed element to the movements. Loading up too many repetitions is a recipe for disaster, especially if you are concerned about adding bulk. Drifting to 8, 10, or 12 reps of moderately heavy weight is the catalyst for growth, so keep the repetitions under 6. (Later in this chapter, we'll revisit the best ways for sets and reps to progress.)

PHASE III | Race–Season Performance

Maintain joint and musculoskeletal integrity and health
Improve muscular power and force potential
Maintain muscular strength
Transfer specific movement patterns into sport-specific movements and power

You will now be well into the racing season, with a few early-season races under your belt, but you won't be hitting those key A races quite yet. It is now time to use the strength gains of the previous two phases to sharpen and refine your skills for racing! There are multiple focus points in this final phase of the year, and you can probably guess that this is the phase where many athletes drop the program altogether, diminishing any opportunity for real benefits.

The omnipresent mobility and stability exercises continue, but there is a radical drop-off in the number of key exercises in this part of the program.

These key exercises all comprise big movements that are an amalgamation of many of the smaller patterns deployed earlier in the program. It is important to maintain the strength gained previously, so the load is high in these key exercises, but the actual weight may well be reduced. Nearly all of the focus is on moving the load *quickly or explosively*. There is plenty of ballistic work, including tossing, jumping, leaping, and driving, all of which leverage previously earned strength and now ask for power. These ballistic movements will help rev up your body and brain for race week.

In addition to this focus, we truly need to maintain musculoskeletal health in this part of the season. I like athletes to have a large focus on overall health and minimizing the damage caused by racing. Carefully monitor your fatigue and performance levels, incorporate a deeper focus on recovery modalities and mobility, and guard against signs of tiredness. You don't want to create a reservoir of fatigue in this part of the season. Instead, aim to stay sharp, fresh, and powerful. This is where you draw from the foundational bank account created by the hard work earlier in the progression. Strength training is still considered to be a key workout during the training week throughout this phase.

We are not aiming to gain big strength here, or to teach ourselves more movement patterns. We are simply aiming to be ready to race well. Don't make the mistake of thinking that power and explosive qualities don't have their place in endurance sports! Of course, we don't want to lose any of the strength gains we have already made, so there is also a strength maintenance element, but that element comes from the large movements included in the program.

DESIGNING A PROGRESSIVE PROGRAM

Bear in mind that strength training cannot be bolted on to your endurance training. This is why I count it among the pillars of performance, with each pillar bearing equal emotional importance. Training is not simply swimming, biking, and running; it is those three disciplines woven into the fabric of recovery, nutrition, and strength. We need to design a strength plan with the other pillars in mind, as well as the rest of your life outside triathlon. Here are some must-have components of your strength program.

The program must be progressive. Begin with the fundamentals, and progress from there. The same session, repeated each week, has very limited long-term value. A point of clarification: Within any specific phase or focus, you can certainly repeat the same session as long as the load, intensity, and/or volume are transforming. Never repeat a session for more than 4 to 6 weeks in a row without changing up the exercises or the actual session structure. Without changes, adaptations will slow. Later in this chapter we will take a closer look at how exercises, as well as sets and reps, progress over the course of strength training.

The program must parallel the endurance season. The progression of the plan must fit within the scope of your overall season and ensure that you are primed for your best performance at the right time. Random strength training and prefabricated programs won't cut it; you must align your strength training with the progression of the overall plan. Table 5.1 shows a typical season progression of swim-bike-run training emphasis coupled with the parallel progression of functional strength training. Your own seasonal progression will need to be adapted to fit your needs and key racing plans.

The program must be easy to integrate into weekly training. It must fit seamlessly within endurance training, so it should be planned for, just like a swim, bike, or run session. Keep your hard days hard and your easy days easy—this is why we usually aim to integrate a strength workout into a training day with a key workout. Functional strength completed on a rest day compromises the ability to truly rest. At the same time, a strength workout with a heavy lower-body load on the same day as a higher-intensity running session can certainly increase the risk of injury; hence, a commonsense approach to integration is important.

The program must be relatively simple. While there are many exercises out there that could benefit you, we have to ensure that the program doesn't take up much time and isn't overly complex. Variety is key, but you shouldn't expect to spend 90 minutes in a functional strength session. I see high yield from regular sessions of 20 to 40 minutes. Of course, this shorter time range makes it easier to combine strength with an endurance session for busy athletes.

The program must be specific enough to actually help performance. While it should be simple, we want all exercises to contribute specifically to your overall performance goals. Beauty in simplistic specifics is the goal.

Experience Counts

Before beginning a program, take the time to reflect and assess your experience and history in strength training. I have met many athletes with a vast amount of endurance experience but a much lower "training age" when it comes to strength training. In fact, some of my professional athletes have evolved to a high level before even applying real strength to their programs. This makes them elite in triathlon but pure juniors in strength.

Your experience level is an important consideration when beginning a plan. If you have little control of your body, or ability to perform the most basic strength exercises, then you should start with the basics and err on the side of being too easy. It takes time to develop competency in the weight room. Athletes who came to triathlon after participating in other sports may find this

TABLE 5.1 | **OVERVIEW OF A TYPICAL SEASON**

SPORT-SPECIFIC TRAINING	MONTH*	FUNCTIONAL STRENGTH TRAINING
Post-season	Oct.	**PHASE I** Foundational Strength & Stability
	Nov.	
	Dec.	
Pre-season Conditioning	Jan.	
	Feb.	**PHASE II** Synchronization & Power
	Mar.	
Sustainable Power & Early Racing	Apr.	
	May	
Main Racing	June	**PHASE III** Race-Season Performance
	July	
	Aug.	
	Sept.	
	Oct.	

*For athletes in the Northern Hemisphere

Note: Don't confuse this progression with classic periodization—the start of a new phase is not a radical departure from the work that came before it. In progressive training the focus of training evolves more fluidly over the course of the season.

type of work significantly easier and experience rewards more quickly than experienced triathletes, thanks to their broader athletic background.

The end goal is to obtain the benefits that real strength provides, but there are no shortcuts. Start from where you are currently, and work steadily. Just as you cannot truly evolve your swimming, biking, and running in one season, the same applies for strength. Keep the long-term goal in mind—you have more than a single season of planning to reach your goals. Getting started is the most important part.

Exercise Progressions

One of the most intimidating components of starting into strength work is the sheer number of exercises to choose from. There are literally thousands of exercises, most of which have multiple variations based on different coaching preferences, desired outcomes, required modifications for particular athletes, and so forth. Here's the dirty secret: *The exercises themselves don't matter all that much.* Working toward the goal of becoming a stronger, more resilient, more athletic triathlon machine is what matters. Exactly how you get to your goal—that is, the exercises you choose to do—is less important.

To illustrate what a progressive functional strength program looks like, we've included sample main sets from each phase of training. (All of these exercises along with some additional dynamic warm-up exercises and ancillary exercises are described in Appendix B.) It would be easy to focus on these individual exercises and simply follow them as your program; however, it's unlikely that it would be the ideal program for you. Some of the exercises we've selected were chosen to illustrate specific concepts, some were adapted to accommodate our model's movement deficits, and others are included simply because they're universally recognized.

The best way to review the three functional strength sessions is to consider the concepts that each exercise illustrates and how the overall program builds strength and resiliency. In fact, these samples don't fully outline the programs that my athletes use. When put into practice, these sample sessions would alternate with a second session that meets the goals for that particular phase.

From Phase I to Phase III, the exercises move from simple to complex, isolated to coordinated, and (in many cases) lower to higher intensity. Throwing a medicine ball over your shoulder may look cool, but before you pick up that ball we need to make sure you can properly stabilize your core and coordinate the movement from the ground through your shoulders. After we take a look at these snapshots of the phases of functional strength training, we will follow one progression through a season so you can get a sense of the bigger picture.

Each exercise in this Phase I session fits a specific category or need based on this athlete's strengths and weakness (Figure 5.1). The exercises are simple, and there is a strong emphasis on reacquiring the ability to move well after a long triathlon season. The main set is broken up to make sure we address the upper body, lower body, and core with both strength and stability exercises.

FIGURE 5.1 | PHASE I SAMPLE SESSION, MAIN SET

DYNAMIC EXERCISE/ EARLY POWER	Propulsions Above Knee 3 × 8	
LOWER-BODY STRENGTH	Medicine-Ball Squats 3 × 10	
LOWER-BODY MOBILITY	Kneeling Hip Extensions 1 × 10 (bilateral)	
UPPER-BODY STRENGTH	Push-ups, wide 3 × 10	

UPPER-BODY MOBILITY	Wall Angels 1 × 10	
STABILITY/ MOBILITY FILLER	Side Planks 1 × 10 (bilateral)	
SECONDARY LOWER-BODY STRENGTH	Front Lunges 3 × 10	
SECONDARY LOWER-BODY MOBILITY	Face-the-Wall Squats 1 × 10	
SECONDARY UPPER-BODY STRENGTH	Seated Rows 3 × 10	
SECONDARY UPPER-BODY MOBILITY	Rib Rolls 1 × 10 (bilateral)	
SECONDARY STABILITY/ MOBILITY FILLER	Quadruped Hip Flexions/ Extensions 1 × 10	

Note: *Functional strength workouts should begin with a proper warm-up. Appendix B includes exercises that work well as dynamic warm-ups.*

This work sets the table for the next phase, where the early regional strength and mobility elements come together in a more complex environment, often combining two of the earlier categories into a single exercise (Figure 5.2). For example, Front Squats are great for lower-body strength development, but they also provide a huge core stability challenge, allowing us to accomplish more in one move. You can see how the exercises in Phase II have evolved from Phase I.

FIGURE 5.2 | **PHASE II SAMPLE SESSION, MAIN SET**

DYNAMIC EXERCISE/ POWER	Propulsions Below Knee 2–3 × 6–8	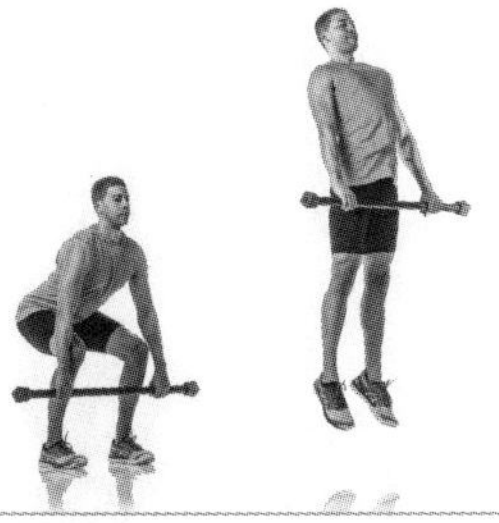
LOWER-BODY STRENGTH	Front Squats 2–3 × 6–8	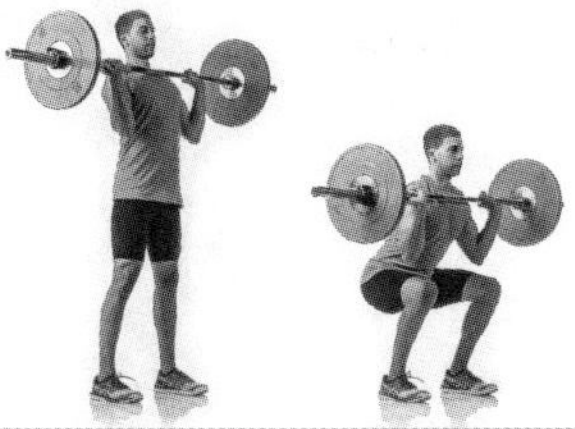
LOWER-BODY POWER	Tuck Jumps with Arms 2–3 × 5	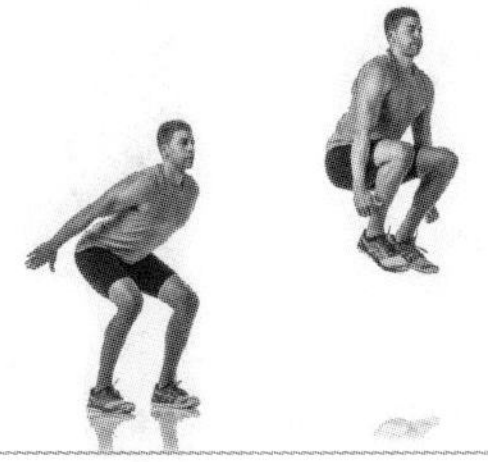
MOBILITY/ STABILITY	Goblet Ride-Downs with Reach 1 × 10	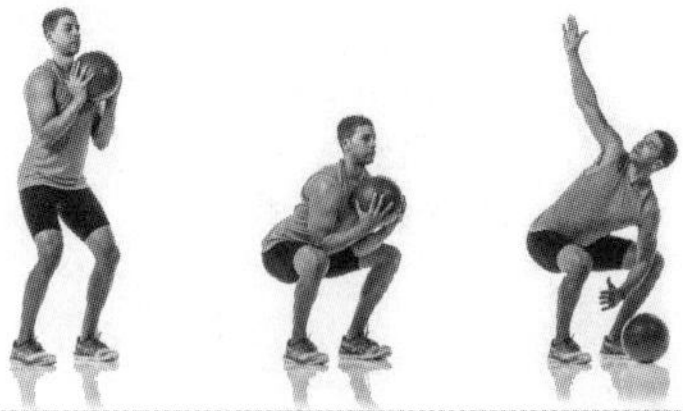

UPPER-BODY STRENGTH	Standing Shoulder Presses 2–3 × 5	
UPPER-BODY STABILITY	Antirotation Punches 2–3 × 6–8	
MOBILITY/ STABILITY	Y's, T's, W's 1 × 10	
LOWER-BODY SINGLE LEG	Step-ups with weight 2–3 × 6–8	

Moving into the race-ready phase of strength training, you can see another round of subtle changes to the programming (Figure 5.3). The goal of this phase is to stay fresh and healthy and get ready to race. Consequently, the volume and duration of the session are significantly reduced, while the intensity is increased. The exercises in Phase III require quicker, more complex movements—often combining what was previously achieved in two or three parts, or exercises, into a whole-body movement.

FIGURE 5.3 | PHASE III SAMPLE FUNCTIONAL STRENGTH SESSION, MAIN SET

UPPER-BODY POWER	Push Jerks 2–3 × 5	
LB UPPER-BODY STRENGTH/ MOBILITY	Y's, T's, W's with bands 2 × 10–15	
POWER (LOWER BODY, CORE, UPPER BODY)	Front Squat to Push Presses 2–3 × 5	
LOWER-BODY STRENGTH/ BALANCE	Single-Leg Romanian Deadlifts 3 × 6–8	
POWER	Scoop Tosses 2 × 3–5	

LOWER-BODY POWER	Dynamic Step-ups 2–3 × 6	

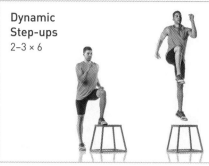

Let's consider how the exercises in Phase III demonstrate the progression to whole-body movements. The Front Squat to Push Presses build upon the improvements in body movements/sequencing that were earned in the earlier weeks with propulsions. The Y's, T's, W's now have a strength component to tackle postural strength, upper-body strength, and mobility in a single exercise. The Single-Leg Romanian Deadlifts maintain earlier strength gains while incorporating a balance component. The road map for your own progressive strength plan should demonstrate gradually increasing challenges, moving from more isolated work to ensure that you have adequate ability in the parts before working on the whole.

Now let's consider a full progression through all the phases of strength training (Figure 5.4). There are many exercises that could prepare you to do a medicine-ball toss, but what follows is the progression we chose and the rationale behind it. For some athletes, this progression would occur over the course of several weeks, while for others, it could take several months. Some athletes will never have to progress past the early steps to reap benefits.

Your own functional strength program should take into account your experience with strength training, your athletic background, and your injury history. The sessions outlined here do not represent the whole plan for any individual athlete. In addition to the strength session, we would include sport-specific drills (such as high knees for running, rolling exercises for swimming, specific power sessions on the bike) and ancillary exercises to address functional and core stability deficits identified in the functional strength assessment found at the end of the chapter—ankle mobility, rotational core stability, and so forth. More emphasis is given to addressing limitations early in the process. In the middle phases of strength training, more sport-specific components are introduced to carry over to the race-ready phase.

FIGURE 5.4 | **FULL PROGRESSION OF PHASES**

PHASE I

Side Planks

Side Clams

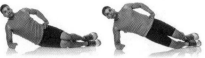 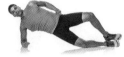

FOUNDATIONAL STRENGTH & STABILITY

Begin with heavy work on lower-body mobility (Kneeling Hip Extensions and Face-the-Wall Squats, Figure 5.1) and core strength (Side Planks). These exercises develop the strength and stability that will protect the spine and create mobility through the hips, which will be required in Phase III.

PHASE II

Antirotation Punches

Standing Contralateral Punches

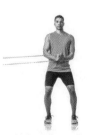 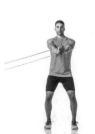 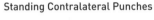 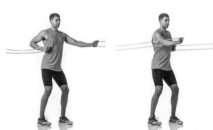

SYNCHRONIZATION & POWER

These exercises challenge the core while standing, first in a basic movement (Antirotation Punches) and then with a more complex challenge (Standing Contralateral Punches). This phase also incorporates Tuck Jumps and Front Squats (Figure 5.2), which are designed to build the ability to produce force from the ground. These exercises are more dynamic and challenging yet still targeted.

Scoop Tosses

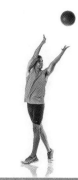

RACE-SEASON PERFORMANCE

Exercise intensity increases in Phase III as frequency and volume decrease. Complex movements that provide overlapping benefits are aimed as much at revving up your nervous system as at improving strength. The progression finishes with the Scoop Tosses.

Progression of Sets and Reps

A truly effective functional strength program is not as simple as something written on an index card and repeated over and over. The focus and emphasis of the training need to progress, and we must synchronize the focus with the progression of our training and racing season. We've illustrated the way different exercises create progression, but as you can imagine, the number of sets and repetitions, as well as the amount of rest, also plays an important role. We want to maximize the benefits of the program without adding much (if any) muscle mass or bulk.

In Phase I you can complete most of the exercises in a circuit—finishing a single set of one exercise and moving to the next, returning to the first exercise only after you have completed each of the exercises on the list. There is little need for much rest between exercises due to the circuit. Because we are focused on establishing efficient movement patterns, you can complete up to 12 repetitions. As soon as you progress to adding load or weight to the exercises, you want to add enough load to ensure that you feel stress by 5 or 6 repetitions. Avoid repetitions of 9 to 14, as this will tend to add muscle mass without proper strength gains. If 5 or 6 repetitions can be completed with ease, check to be sure you are completing the exercise correctly and not cheating yourself. It could be the case that you need to add more load or complexity to the exercise. There is little value in completing high repetitions with lower weight. All that said, there's one principle that dictates our decision-making process when it comes to functional strength training: *form over force.*

As we progress through Phase II and Phase III, the stress and load go up, but the number of exercises drops. In this phase you will only want to complete 3 to 6 repetitions of the key exercises, with plenty of rest between exercises. You can supplement the rest time with ancillary exercises that don't target the muscles you just placed under load. Feel free to continue with the circuit format, but each key exercise must be completed fresh, following rest. This means you will need to take several minutes before repeating a key set.

It's easy to see why many athletes disregard functional strength training. To do it correctly, you need to make a concerted effort. Here are the takeaways I hope to leave you with:

- Functional strength training is an important and necessary component of triathlon training.
- Functional strength training should complement, not replace, your training.
- There is no one-size-fits-all approach, especially with regard to beginning a program.
- A good program is progressive, both during the season and over the course of multiple seasons.
- Simply starting a progressive program is most important.

FUNCTIONAL STRENGTH SELF-ASSESSMENT

The final piece of the puzzle is a series of assessments to help guide your path and focus. Keep in mind that these assessments are evaluations, not tests that you pass or fail. You may never "pass" the lat test, for example, for a host of reasons (such as previous injury or genetics)—but improvement is still beneficial. The assessments are especially important as you start a program, as they can help you identify specific weaknesses and issues that are either areas of potential injury or ongoing limiters on your improvement of biomechanics or power production. These are some common problems that triathletes face. If you identify an area of weakness or reduced range of motion, take note of the specific exercises and interventions that will help you build strength or improve mobility in that area.

Thoracic Spine (Midback) & Shoulder

This is a common area of weakness and lack of mobility in many athletes, and the problem is heightened for those who spend time in front of the computer or have extensive cycling background. Thoracic mobility and shoulder function go hand in hand. Poor thoracic/shoulder performance can affect the ability to achieve proper extension and shoulder rotation in the pool and may lead to the injury known as swimmer's shoulder. It also has an effect on the ability to hold proper postural integrity in the time trial position on the bike.

WALL ANGELS TEST

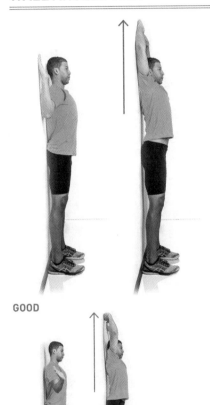

GOOD

POOR

Stand with your heels, midback, and back of your head against a wall. Make big "snow angels," keeping your hands as close to the wall as possible. You should be able to perform the motion without your arms pulling away from the wall and without losing good posture.

Potential problem areas: Thoracic mobility, shoulder mobility, computer posture (extending head out in front of the chest)

Interventions: Rib Rolls (p. 312); Y's, T's, W's (p. 315); Wall Angels (p. 310); thoracic mobility drills

Shoulder Mobility

We want to get more specific on shoulder mobility and range of motion around the joint. Apart from playing a contributing role in the time trial position, the lats are the biggest source of power potential in swimming. Without proper mobility, you will never be able to gain full power potential from the pull phase of the swimming stroke.

LAT TEST

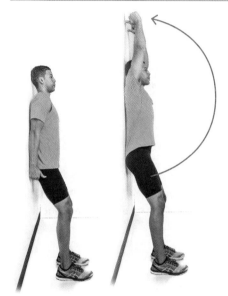

Half squat with your back against the wall; keep the elbows straight, and reach up, trying to touch the wall above your head.

Potential problem areas: Shoulder mobility, especially lats, which are a common cause of weakness and low mobility for triathletes

Interventions: Mobility exercises; long pulling exercises (full body chops/lifts)

EXCELLENT
Touch wall

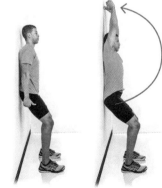

POOR
Uneven, unable to touch the wall

Lumbar Spine

The lumbar spine is a key anchor for all three disciplines in triathlon and a common area of weakness and low mobility. Cycling creates huge postural stress on the lumbar region (especially the discs), especially when followed by the jarring of running. A stable core makes for a powerful engine, so this area is key for performance—especially considering the fact that you must be able to run well immediately after finishing the bike portion of a triathlon.

LOWER-BACK ENDURANCE TEST

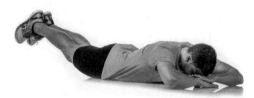

GOOD
80 seconds female
100 seconds male

Lying on firm ground, stack your hands on the ground to support your forehead. Keeping your legs straight, lift both legs off the ground. Make sure your knees clear the floor. Stop the test when fatigue makes either or both knees touch the floor.

Potential problem areas: Lumbar endurance

Interventions: Switch "core work" to focus more on low-back and side stabilizers.

Note: The times given are the minimum acceptable for triathletes in my experience (and differ from clinical back-pain models).

Hip and Lower Extremities

This is a key area of identification of hip and lower extremity power production. The aim is to identify and develop a hip-squatting form, as moving through the hip is powerful. Once you are able to drive through the hips, that movement translates into bike and run power potential and the ability to maintain stable hips during both activities.

FACE-THE-WALL SQUAT TEST

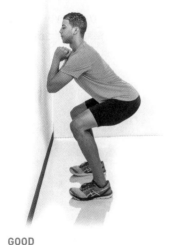

GOOD

Starting about 12 inches away from the wall, drop down into a squat.

Potential problem areas: If you find that your knees are hitting the wall, you're not taking full advantage of your hips as a power generator.

Interventions: Use this test to build range of motion. To improve glute strength, use Goblet Ride-Downs with Reach (p. 314), other hip mobility exercises, and Step-ups (p. 325).

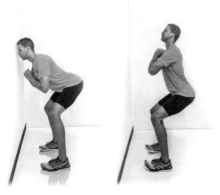

POOR
Falling forward   *Falling back*

Balance/Stability

This assessment identifies issues with central nervous system control and balance/strength. Is your brain talking to your muscles? Muscles are only as good as their connections—strong muscles that respond late don't help. These areas have a huge correlation with bike and run performance.

SINGLE-LEG BALANCE TEST

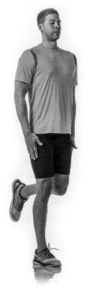

GOOD
Minimum of at least 20 seconds before failure

Standing on one leg with your eyes open, fix your gaze straight ahead and close your eyes.

Potential problem areas: balance, motor control

Interventions: balance work, single-leg stance work

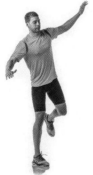

FAILURE
Foot touching support leg, hopping, using arms for balance

Ankle Mobility

Poor ankle mobility contributes to many lower-leg injuries as well as limited run biomechanics. Some limited evidence indicates that this test may actually predict injury. Stiffness in the ankle joint necessitates compensation that often leads to injury.

WALL TEST (modified lunge test)

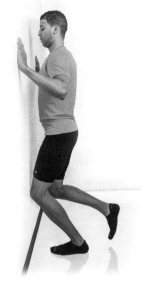

Starting with the toes of one foot touching the wall, push your knee forward to touch the wall. Keep moving your foot backward until you can no longer touch the wall with your knee. Mark the spot. Repeat on the opposite leg.

Potential problem areas: ankle mobility

Interventions: stretching, mobility work for the calf/ankle region

EXCELLENT
>2 inches from wall

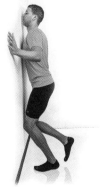

POOR
<1 inch from wall

part II

ENDURANCE TRAINING

6

Swimming in Triathlon

The expression on the faces of competitors at the start line of a triathlon says it all: "Get me on my bike." The swim portion of the race can elicit great fear and anxiety about being ill-prepared to face a cluster of thrashing bodies in a radically dynamic environment. It's an ominous scene marked by a frightening reality: Most triathletes don't have the training, skills, or specific preparation to manage and truly race this portion of the triathlon. For most of us, the swim is a necessary evil standing between us and the rest of the race.

Many athletes struggle to make meaningful gains in swimming and resign themselves to the fact that they are simply "poor swimmers." As a result, they place more of their focus on preparing for the other two disciplines. Others don't try to justify a lopsided approach; they simply don't have additional time to dedicate to swimming while maintaining cycling and running training. Whatever the story, many triathletes simply don't put in enough swim training time to see great results.

Those athletes who remain committed to improvement across all three sports often fall prey to a massive push of education and information promoting a swimming technique that doesn't work for triathlon. Enticed by promises of "shortcuts to success," they focus too heavily on technique over consistent, strong, and specific prescriptions of conditioning, and the very metrics they use to improve their stroke actually hold them back. The swim lanes are full of swimmers doing drills that look pretty, but they fall short of their goals on race day.

When they aren't doing drills, most triathletes are swimming up and down the pool to accumulate a certain time or distance or joining masters classes or group sessions focused on pool swimming. Many are missing the variety that maximizes positive adaptations as well as specific preparation for their races, most of which are held in open water.

As I see it, many triathletes adopt an approach to swimming that devalues training time, focuses on technical improvements over conditioning, and lacks specific preparation. The end result is that athletes are training too little and too slow without the appropriate focus on the specific demands of the event. These three issues lead to an ongoing cycle of frustration for many triathletes. It is no wonder that so many become resigned to maintaining their current level of performance. After all, their training isn't providing results.

As a former elite swimmer, an NCAA Division I swimming coach, and a front-of-the-pack swimmer in my professional racing, I am passionate about the swimming portion of triathlon. However, once I became a coach for the sport, I had to undergo a real education in the specifics of triathlon swimming. I quickly realized that the sport has many athletes who are in different stages of development and have very different goals. All of my swim coaching had been done with swimmers, and I soon became aware that what is appropriate for an ex–elite swimmer is very different than what is required for most triathletes. Over the past 10 years of coaching, I have begun to understand the rift that separates classical swimming training from open-water performance. There are many differences, beginning with technique and extending to the workout progression and specificity that come with triathlon racing. I spent a lot of time talking with other athletes and coaches about swimming: the role it plays in overall performance, how it should be approached, and how to make it a gateway to improved biking and running performance. Ultimately, I came to the realization that we need to change the way we approach triathlon swimming.

We will meet the challenge head-on in this chapter by finding a clear and smart path forward and identifying a better way to structure training. I can say with confidence that this approach will yield speed and performance gains that will pay off come race day.

DEBUNKING THE MYTHS OF TRIATHLON SWIMMING

The concept of the importance of the swim is slowly gaining traction in mainstream triathlon, but there are plenty of common (and corrosive) myths about triathlon swimming that get in the way of our progress. In fact, you may have expected to see some of the following ideas and directives in the how-to section. If you can turn your back on the false promises promoted by these ideas, I am confident that you can become a better swimmer.

MYTH: **Additional swim training is not a good use of training time.** Many athletes believe that because the swim is the shortest leg of the race, we should spend less time training for it. This is the biggest myth of all. Triathlon swimming is a part of a sport that is swim-bike-run, and the effects of each discipline are felt throughout overall performance. The lessons and physical benefits of a balanced approach will be explored in this chapter, and I'm confident that you won't regret investing some more time in your swim training.

MYTH: **Higher distance per stroke is the key to speed.** By far the most prevalent approach to "stroke improvement" is an effort to decrease the number of strokes in each lap. The logic is that the fewer strokes you take, the more efficient you are, and being more efficient must be better! This thinking has led to the proliferation of triathletes with very long strokes; very slow turnover; and, by extension, longer swim splits. Eliminating stroke rate from the performance equation is ludicrous, yet that's exactly what most triathletes do when they set out to improve their freestyle stroke.

MYTH: **Focus on rotation and gliding.** Reduction of drag is always a good thing, but developmental swimmers tend to give it far too much emphasis. Like the fixation on distance per stroke, a singular focus on getting "thin," extending the glide, or reducing drag can lead to unintended consequences. Trying to mimic what Michael Phelps looks like underwater won't make you a better swimmer. I see too many swimmers rolling onto their side and gliding like a long, thin sailboat. They do manage to reduce drag, but they aren't moving forward very fast. Why is this? It's simple—propulsion! Most developmental swimmers lack a strong, propulsive kick and specific muscular power and endurance, and they will never develop that kick if they focus on gliding through the water. Sure, a long stroke with a delayed catch is effective for

DISTANCE PER STROKE: WHY LONGER IS NOT BETTER

Because swimming is generally less familiar than cycling and running, let's use a running analogy to explore why fewer strokes might not be the best approach to swimming. Imagine I asked you to run around a track at a moderate effort and count your steps over the 400 meters. Let's say it took you 2 minutes and 180 steps to complete the lap, or 90 steps each minute (counting one leg only). This is a good foot speed for runners.

Next I tell you to run another 400 meters, and this time I want you to take fewer steps—after all, the fewer steps you take, the more efficient you will be. To compensate, you lengthen your stride considerably and manage to get down to 170 steps, or 85 steps per minute. Have you become a better runner? We cannot answer that question without knowing how quickly you took those steps. Chances are very good that you are not a better runner—now you just overstride, which likely means you are running a little slower.

The analogy doesn't fit perfectly, as we are exerting force against very different mediums in running (air) and swimming (water), but the basic concept is the same. Running speed is an index of the distance of your stride × the number of strides taken over a set time. The same applies in swimming. Water is a very-high-density medium that retards speed more than air does. It takes very specific muscular power and endurance to overcome this effect. A weaker swimmer will experience high peaks and valleys of velocity, often exaggerated by a long stroke and a weak kick, a combination that results in major deceleration. A focus on stroke rate will prevent such large decelerations and allow the swimmer to maintain speed. We then simply need to train the endurance and power (propulsion) to improve sustainable speed.

the best swimmers, such as Michael Phelps. But they also rely on a massive "motorboat" kick, which prevents deceleration at any phase of the stroke, and they deploy these strengths strategically in events that are typically just minutes long. By contrast, if you have an ineffective kick, then the extended pause (which is common in what is often called "front-quadrant swimming") will only lead to a drop in body position and to slowing. This technique simply is not useful for swimmers who race in the open-water environment because they need to make a fast transition from entry to propulsion and hence need a higher stroke rate.

MYTH: **Smart drills make a faster swimmer.** Drills focus on a small piece of the stroke with the hope that breaking the stroke down into sections and then gradually putting the sections back together will help the athlete become a better overall swimmer. While drills can effectively create improvement in certain situations, their value is grossly overestimated, especially when the swimmer lacks wherewithal, or the necessary foundation. Let's consider the typical scenario: Most triathletes get to swim two to five times each week; elite athletes fit in more swim workouts if they have the time. This is not a huge amount of swimming time relative to what athletes who compete only as swimmers would accomplish in a week. It's my experience that a cost-benefit analysis of integrating more drills shows that they rarely translate to improved swimming for triathletes. If you are a budding triathlete swimmer, here is the headline: *Use the majority of your time in the pool to develop adequate conditioning and for focused, specific training.* You will be better off if you integrate technical focus into the actual swimming session and utilize specific tools (or toys, as we like to call them) that will assist with the adoption of proper form while also improving fitness and endurance.

Swimming is a technical sport, and drills and technical work are well worth the time in competitive swimming, when the events last 20 seconds to 15 minutes and you have many sessions and hours each week to apply appropriate focus to the fine points of technique.

MYTH: **Long and easy steady-state training unlocks swim performance.** My local pool is regularly filled with triathletes accumulating lap after lap of steady-state swimming to hit a set time or distance. If you are serious about improving your performance in the triathlon swim, there is little to no value in extended slow swimming, especially if you are relatively new to the sport. Nearly all of your sessions should be broken into interval-based swimming to ensure that you can maintain good form at a speed that will elicit improvements. This is not to say that all of your swimming sessions should consist of short, hard efforts. Endurance work is of critical value to all athletes, but I am opposed to unstructured sessions at a fixed pace. Any session for the two-swims-per-week triathlete prescribed as "30 minutes smooth steady-state" has low value relative to more targeted prescriptions of speed variance and may even be detrimental.

MYTH: **There's a limit to how much your swimming will improve.** There is a pervasive belief in some quarters of triathlon that unless you grew up swimming, it is impossible to progress very far in the sport. This simply isn't true, and it further reflects the way swim training is undervalued within the sport. If you are patient, are willing to do the work, and structure the seasonal training appropriately, you can make great gains. The tough reality is that it typically takes a long time to evolve as a triathlete swimmer, even with the proper prescription, in just a few swim sessions each week. Give it time, and results will come from great consistency in both effort and application.

A NEW APPROACH TO TRIATHLON SWIMMING

If we view triathlon as three distinct sports linked together over the course of racing, we will approach training and technique for swimming, cycling, and running as mutually exclusive events. This might work in training, but on race day it is impossible to segregate the three sports.

Triathlon is not swimming, biking, and running—it is swim-bike-run. One sport completed in that order on race day. What happens during the cycling portion of the race can certainly be influenced by the swim, and what happens during the run can absolutely be influenced by both the swimming and cycling that preceded the final segment. This is how any athlete who is serious about improvements over the long term should view the sport of triathlon. We are not swimmers, cyclists, and runners—we are *triathletes.* We need to train for the sport of triathlon, and the swim is an all-important discipline that sets the tone for the rest of the day.

This is the framework for how we will train for swimming, approach racing, and develop a performance mind-set, and we will use the same framework for cycling and running. We are not training for swimming; we are not even training for open-water racing. We are training for an open-water race that is followed by cycling and running. Many athletes and coaches forget this simple fact and justify their inadequate attention to swimming as a part of their overall plan. How often do you hear it said that because the swim makes up a smaller percentage of the race compared to the bike and the run, it's better to invest more training in the other disciplines? Don't underestimate the importance of swimming. Cultivate a willingness to put in the time and effort required to evolve in this portion of triathlon. In order to truly change, athletes and coaches must collectively acknowledge that preparation and training for swimming is equal in value to the other two disciplines. It's my hope that you will be open to shifting your focus as a swimmer.

BENEFITS OF IMPROVED SWIMMING

The good news is that the benefits of better swimming extend well beyond the minute or two that you will pick up in your race splits.

Fitness overflow. From a musculoskeletal standpoint, swimming is the least corrosive discipline. This advantage allows for massive fitness gains over the course of your training program that carry over to the other disciplines. I am not suggesting that you can become "bike-ready" or "run-ready" by simply swimming, but swim training is a good supporting player in the pursuit of cardiovascular conditioning. It is worth mentioning that athletes tend to be able to hit higher intensity more frequently in swimming as a result of the reduced muscular impact. It's yet another aspect of improved cardiovascular conditioning for swim-fit athletes to enjoy.

Reduced energy cost. Much of triathlon racing success is about pacing your effort throughout the race to maintain effort and output in the run, the last third of the race. This requires appropriate effort and pacing across all three sports. Specific training, accompanied by solid fitness, enables you to expend less energy in finishing the initial portion. Beyond the physical demands of race day, I believe you have to dose your willpower—after all, we do not have an endless reserve. Arriving swim-ready means that the swim portion demands less emotional energy, meaning it has become more automatic and thus leaves more willpower, or emotional reserves, for pushing yourself when it really counts. It is virtually impossible to separate the physical from the emotional, so swim preparedness undoubtedly minimizes the overall energy cost on race day.

A good school of learning. Nearly all of your swimming will be done in a controlled environment—the swimming pool! You have flat water; a set distance for each lap; and ongoing feedback, thanks to the pace clock. This makes swim training the perfect opportunity to learn pacing, perceived effort, and the relationship between shifting effort and increasing speed. Athletes who grew up in competitive swimming have an unparalleled sense of pacing and timing as well as a strong internal sense of rate of perceived effort. Learning to feel pace and exertion is quite often a challenge for athletes, and there is no better way to develop this ability than through consistent swimming. As you develop this feedback loop, it becomes much easier to transfer the lessons to other sports, such as cycling and running, which typically take place in more dynamic environments. I sometimes refer to swim sessions as a chance to experience risk-free failure. Pace a session poorly, and you will suffer. Go out too hard in the initial 100 yards of a 500-yard effort, and you will suffer. The feedback loop is there, if you are listening. Take advantage of the opportunity—stay mentally engaged throughout your training sessions, and perform the types of sessions required to provide this kind of learning.

The value of practice over perfection. There is little doubt that a commitment to improved swimming entails patience, planning, commitment to long-term development, seasonal progression, and more. This seemingly myopic commitment has the potential to expand every athlete's vision of what it takes to succeed both in the sport and in other areas of life. In many ways, it's like learning to paint. Many people claim they cannot paint, but the truth is that anyone can learn. It is no different than any other pursuit (coding, playing a musical instrument, picking up a new language) that initially feels foreign. Natural ability may separate us from the real experts, but, as a friend of mine is quick to say, learning to paint is simply about overcoming our inhibitions about painting. I encourage you to bring the same mentality to improving your swim. If you focus on the practice of swimming and not on perfection, you will find it more rewarding.

Student of tactics. In addition to improving our physical ability to swim, we can learn how to respond to the dynamic open-water environment. Tactical acumen will lead to improved performance in triathlon swimming—learning the influence of waves, sun, gear changes (swim speed), and other competitors, all while holding a straight line! Become a student of tactics, and you will become a better open-water swimmer, saving energy and maximizing speed in the swim. In addition to all of this, you will certainly be making a huge deposit to your confidence.

Because of all of these benefits, it's been my experience that when athletes work on their swimming, they become better athletes in the other two sports as well. I have never seen an athlete regress as a triathlete because of a focus on swimming. I have only seen 100 percent progression. So, whatever the cause, it seems that there is good reason to apply yourself in the pool under proper guidance and with the correct training prescription.

TECHNICAL FOUNDATIONS

My goal is to outline the key aspects to consider and focus on within your triathlon swim training. It is important to realize that as a triathlete (especially at the longer distances), you are an open-water swimmer, and that this is very different from competitive pool swimming. For the same reason that we wouldn't model your running form for an Ironman race after Usain Bolt, there is no use in trying to learn technical improvements by watching Michael Phelps. Triathlon swimming is a different sport, at a different level, with different requirements.

What follows is informed by my belief that for most triathletes, the technical focus of swimming is overexaggerated, as we explored earlier in this chapter. The real route to improvement, given time constraints, is to get the basics of the stroke as close to correct as possible, then apply specific, progressive, and consistent load for an extended period. When a few stroke fundamentals are established and supported with consistent training, the mechanics of the stroke will fall into place. In addition, we must then learn and apply specific skills for open-water performance. After all, you will usually race in open water, not in the pool.

Alignment

Make it your goal to have good alignment in your swimming stroke. Imagine a straight line that dissects your body along the center, extending out in front of and behind you. The simple rule is that everything on the right side of the body remains on the right side of the line, whether above or below the water. Everything on the left side of the body therefore remains on that side. There is no crossover—at entry, in propulsive pull, or in the recovery phase of the stroke.

I will add a secondary yet important focus when considering the propulsive pull phase of the stroke. Imagine two further lines that run parallel to the center line but extend within the lines of your shoulders (see Figure 6.1). From hand entry to the point where you "create purchase," or hold on the water, to driving water back in the propulsive pull phase, your hand will always stay on the appropriate side of the center line but within the outside line of the shoulder. Note that your elbow will likely fall outside the shoulder line with the natural internal rotation of the shoulder that causes the elbow to face out.

PRACTICING ALIGNMENT

A snorkel is the optimal tool to assist with learning proper alignment. Because it eliminates the usual head swivel that accompanies the breathing motion, you can increase your focus on swimming with good alignment and see when your alignment is incorrect. As an added benefit, a good triathlon-specific snorkel will ensure that you maintain the appropriate head position. Snorkel drills might be the very best available to developing triathlete swimmers.

Taut Body

The second area of focus is the functional posture of your body. Although many athletes place great emphasis on posture on dry land, they tend to make little of it in the water. A taut body is key to your development as a swimmer. This is a challenging concept for new swimmers because of the sense of water as a foreign environment. Many swimmers "noodle" along in the pool, hips swaying from side to side, creating a cascade of negative reactions. Swimmers need to learn how to *hold their bodies within the swimming stroke*. It is almost like learning how to walk again! There are no drills, except for some early-season vertical kicking in deep water, to help develop better swimming posture—the real route is frequent and ongoing practice. It takes time, but the good news is that you can improve this fundamental skill while working on other performance elements such as fitness or muscular endurance.

FIGURE 6.1 | **PROPER SWIMMING TECHNIQUE**

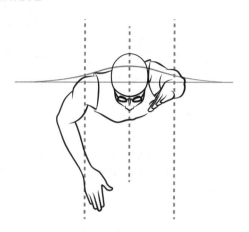

ENTRY

Let the hand drop into the water (avoid mechanically placing it), not at full arm extension but far from the head. The hand should fall between your center line and the outside line of your shoulder without any forceful action. All active effort occurs once the hand is in the water, so the entry is passive and relaxed.

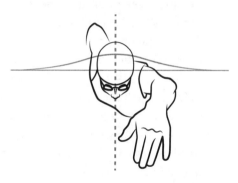

PROPULSIVE PULL

There is no glide in swimming. Once the hand enters, the goal is to "collect" water while achieving a biomechanical position that maximizes the opportunity to push water back, creating propulsion. The pull itself begins with this catch—a smooth motion accelerating to a violent drive of water behind the body. All the while, the hand and arm maintain good purchase on the water, staying inside that same channel from center line to the outside of the shoulder.

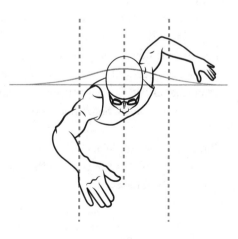

RECOVERY

Finish the pull phase by accelerating water past the hip, then move to the passive, relaxed recovery phase, where the hand transitions from pull exit back to entry. Traditional swimmers will focus on a high elbow and relaxed shoulder-shrug recovery, but this is less important in open-water swimming or for the typical triathlete. Just stay relaxed and leave the active work for when the hand is in the water.

Propulsive Pull

The final element of fundamental mechanics is the pull phase of the stroke. In competitive swimming, this can be a highly technical and analyzed portion of the swimming stroke because very small differences lead to big improvements—or, rather, small changes that are significant! In triathlon swimming, it is absolutely fine to approach this element with a very simple goal. We want to create purchase, or hold, on the water, then push it back behind us with great acceleration. As my former purplepatch pro Luke Bell likes to say, "Grip it and rip it!" As simplistic as this is, if you practice good alignment and posture, then pull does not need to be overcomplicated. Upon entry, the arm and forearm will fall toward the bottom of the pool in a passive collection of water. You can almost imagine collecting water under the armpit. As this entry and collection occur, your palm and forearm will be facing back behind you. In a continuous motion, with no specific glide phase, you then accelerate the hand (and the collected water!) behind you in one continuous and *powerful* movement. Your hand and forearm remain facing back behind you throughout the propulsive pull until water is driven beyond your hip. Think no more about it than this, as the entire pull phase is completed in under a second. Don't complicate it beyond what is necessary.

Beyond these three basic principles of stroke mechanics, we should also include a couple of other specific necessities to improved open-water swimming performance.

Stroke Rate

In the same way that cadence is important in running performance and efficiency, stroke rate is a key element to improving swim performance. If you survey a triathlon swim from a position where you can view the race leaders, the upper-middle pack, the middle pack, and the back of the pack, you might notice some strange swim mechanics within each group, but you will certainly see slower stroke rates as your eyes scan toward the back of the field. Stroke rate, or the number of strokes that you take in a minute, should be balanced with distance per stroke for optimal swimming, but the vast majority of triathletes should prioritize stroke rate over distance per stroke. Yes, we want to move water backward, but we want to do so with a high number of repetitions each minute. This is a skill that is highly trainable yet is often not focused on in training.

In a sport that is often performed in rough conditions and is followed by sports (cycling and running) in which the legs are dominant, it makes perfect sense to develop a higher stroke rate—there's no better way to both save the legs and maximize performance in open water. Ironically, this skill is also employed in competitive swimming. While many elite swimmers look graceful and smooth, their typical stroke rate is much faster than that of most triathletes. It is not uncommon to see triathletes swim with stroke rates of 40, 50, or 60 per minute (one stroke being one single-arm rotation; rotational movement of both the right and left arm is two strokes). The goal should be to progress toward 70, 80, or even 90 strokes per minute. A word of warning, as you cannot simply jump from 45 to 80 strokes per minute and expect great results. You still have to *push water backward*, and you must adapt to a faster stroke turnover, which comes at a greater cardiovascular cost. An incremental increase of 2 percent every few weeks is the best route to improvement.

Another benefit of a higher stroke rate has to do with that oh-so-beneficial thing called oxygen. If you are swimming at 40 strokes per minute and breathing every other stroke (see "Breathing"), then you are going to achieve only 20 breaths within 1 minute of swimming. Increase this to 70 strokes per minute, and you will now have the opportunity to breathe 35 times each minute. To see which is better, I encourage you to run for 5 minutes at a moderately strong effort, but limit yourself to no more than 20 breaths per minute. You will be dying for a break before you know it!

TIP *If stroke rate is an issue for you, a Tempo Trainer (a metronome device that fits under a swim cap) is a wonderful tool that will remind you to maintain a slightly elevated stroke rate.*

Breathing

We can all acknowledge the benefits of breathing. Unfortunately, too many athletes fall into the trap of limiting the number of breaths taken each minute. In some cases, this is the result of a slower stroke rate, but athletes in pursuit of improved technique are often lacking oxygen too. There is an old belief that breathing every third, fourth, or fifth stroke will lead to great efficiency and a smoother stroke. Even if that were the case, the negative effects of not breathing would far outweigh any technical gains. Learn how to integrate breathing into your stroke, then breathe every other stroke throughout training and racing—in other words, every second arm stroke or once every rotational cycle of both arms.

Being able to breathe on both sides is useful in the open-water environment, but let's return to our stroke-rate example above before we jump to conclusions. Imagine that you currently take only 40 strokes each minute but aim to breathe bilaterally, or every third stroke. That would equate to just over 13 breaths per minute. Now, it is time for you to get dressed in your running gear again. . . . I would like you to head out for another 5-minute run at a moderately strong effort. This time I want you to breathe no more than 14 times per minute. Yes, I noticed my generosity there—I could have asked for 13! Let me know how that feels. There is no place in triathlon swimming for breathing every third, fourth, or fifth stroke, especially in main training swim sets or races.

Specific Muscular Endurance and Strength

The final area of focus, which just barely falls into the technical bucket, is the development of specific muscular endurance, strength, and power. This development occurs through consistent and specific swim training, and it should be built on top of the fundamentals mentioned earlier. If you can create a taut body and good alignment, integrate breathing, and move water backward, then your foundation of technical swimming is in place. Now you must learn to improve your swimming-specific muscular power and your muscular endurance to hold that power. This arrives out of consistently strong training and also out of specific training sessions designed to improve these factors. At the end of the chapter, you'll find more detail on specific sessions for each phase of training.

OPEN-WATER SKILLS

Discussions of technical ability in swimming are important, but our sport exists in the dynamic environment of open water. To become a better open-water swimmer, you must consider some of the skills required to be successful in that particular environment and in the swimming pack.

Stroke Changes

You may have to deploy different types of strokes to be successful in open water. It is a dynamic environment, with waves, chop, and rolling tides as well as hundreds of your friends trying to swim over the top of you. Your pretty pool-based swimming technique may not allow for the best progress. You should be able to deploy a higher and straighter arm recovery to avoid chop, and certainly you should employ a faster stroke rate with higher turnover in tough or crowded conditions. Even Michael Phelps would be well served to adapt his beautiful pool-based stroke if he was racing in a crowd and in choppy conditions.

Sighting

Learning how to properly sight, and how often, is critical to successfully navigating a triathlon swim. There are two main considerations:

- How to sight technically
- How and when to sight during a race

Technically, the sight sequence should be integrated into the breathing phase of the stroke. There are variations, but I prefer one specific method. Imagine that you are breathing to your right side. To sight properly, you should lift your

TRIATHLON SWIMMING SQUADS

Your chances of measurable, continued success are greatly improved if you have ongoing access to a high-quality coached swimming environment that focuses on triathlon. Tower 26 (www.tower26.com) in Southern California sets up a progressive swim training program that aligns with a typical triathlon season. Combining multiple pool-based sessions with weekly open-water-specific sessions, it's a beacon of what triathlon swimming programs should be. In San Francisco, our purplepatch triathlon swimming squad takes a similar approach. There are many others, as well as some wonderful group-based options that are not entirely focused on triathlon. Participating in one of these programs provides a fantastic platform for coaching, support, camaraderie, and effective challenge.

Not every athlete will have access to a group like this, but it's possible to work around this lack to ensure that the training you do complete is effective and appropriate for your goals.

If you are an amateur triathlete who is not part of a specific training group, then finding a local masters team or training group is typically beneficial. While you may not achieve the specificity of the key sessions in this group, you will gain from swimming with others at or around your level and be challenged in ways that are impossible to achieve while swimming solo. Even with less specificity, I typically like athletes to supplement their key sessions with group-based swimming.

head up and out of the water so that you can see ahead of you as your left arm begins the recovery part of the stroke (when the left arm is exiting the water). Your mission is then to *look for and see the buoy ahead of you* that you are aiming for as your left arm is recovering. A good tip is to think about taking a quick snapshot of whatever is in front of you that you will process as your head drops back into the water. Within one motion, as you lift, look, and "take a snapshot," you then continue by rotating your head to the right and taking your breath. This is known as the lift-look-and-breathe style, and it should involve minimal disruption in stroke rate or timing. A potential addition that helps some athletes is to think about pressing down with the leading right arm after hand entry, or before the catch as you lift your head.

It is worth noting that a look does not count as a sight. In other words, you get credit for a sight only if you can spot the buoy you are aiming for. If you look ahead and don't see the buoy, then you *continue the sighting sequence until you do.* This reduces the likelihood of heading off course. In a race situation, you should be sighting every sixth stroke or so.

You can also develop other tools to help you with sighting and, hence, swimming in a straight line. First, consider what you are looking for. The immediate target is the buoy, which you hope is in the line you are swimming along. This is your target. There are two other reference points to help you gauge that buoy line. The first is the buoy that you are swimming from, and the other is the coast or shoreline. All three are potential points of reference to assist in navigation. Of course, even with these three points, those pesky little buoys are often tough to spot! I encourage my athletes to always be aware of other, larger landmarks. Is there a peninsula or a set of trees in line with your path? Can you see a hotel on the beach that is in line with the buoys? Such points of reference can keep you generally headed in the right direction. The final reference point might even be the sun, with the understanding that it is gradually going to move in the sky. Of course, we hope you will not be in the water long enough for it to move far.

The Drafting Question

How many triathlete swimmers do you know who are truly accomplished and proficient at open-water swimming and navigation? Perhaps a few of the very top performers, but these are the swimmers whom you would be unlikely to be able to stay with, yes? As I thought, most of your triathlon buddies have pretty poor navigation skills in open water. Guess what? This is typical! For this reason, in the amateur ranks, drafting in open water is vastly overrated as a priority of focus for success. Don't simply think that because you managed to draft in another athlete's wake, you are buying success. You will certainly gain energy-saving benefits (between 3 percent and 7 percent, depending on whether you are drafting on feet or hips), but you will likely be drafting on someone with very poor navigational skills. You may be swimming faster but zigzagging all over the course.

Instead of simply trying to "find feet," I much prefer athletes to retain control and *draft only if the benefit is obvious.* It is more important to swim in a straight line with proper pacing. Get this right first, and you are sure to be

GETTING YOUR SWIM EQUIPMENT RIGHT

While there isn't much equipment in swimming, the choices you do have can dramatically affect your performance, especially on race day. The most basic yet important consideration is your goggles. You should always arrive at a race with a pair of dark or mirrored goggles and also with a pair that has clear or lighter-tinted lenses. You can never predict the conditions, and the appropriate lenses will help keep you on track and swimming in a straight line. Just because they look cool doesn't mean they are the best choice for you. Choose goggles that have a good range of vision and are comfortable and leakproof. You shouldn't need mask-type goggles; you're not going deep-sea diving, and they are too easily pulled off by a straying arm of an unwitting competitor.

The other key equipment choice is your wetsuit. This is a category in which the more expensive suit will not necessarily make you faster. Your wetsuit should be very tight-fitting but should also allow a good range of motion and mobility in the shoulders. For developing swimmers, the cheaper suits are often more appropriate because they tend to have more rigid midsections, hence assisting you to retain a more taut body. The amazing aspect of wetsuits is that the same suit can perform very differently for different swimmers, and the time differences can be significant. In controlled conditions, we have even seen wild speed swings for the same swimmer, and there doesn't seem to be a pattern of fast or slow suits. This is why a controlled test of suits, in a pool, makes for a better purchase.

in a solid place. If you start well, set your pacing properly, and have strong navigational skills, then you can look around you and judge whether there is a slightly faster swimmer whom you can draft from and benefit from being in that person's wake. Even in this situation, don't be a lemming and simply follow the faster swimmer all over the course. Remain aware, sight frequently, and make smart decisions about your direction and course throughout the swim. You can see how skills development and race wisdom are huge components of swim performance. We will take a closer look at pacing and other components of racing in Chapter 11.

TRAINING THE SWIM IN TRIATHLON

When we think about the season progression as a part of triathlon, it is important to remember that we can leverage the three sports. In an increasingly year-round sport, I like athletes to give their musculoskeletal system time to repair and rejuvenate each season. For this reason, I often prescribe a lower total running load in the post-season and pre-season phases, especially in single-session duration. While it is important to maintain some running and to include specific work in that discipline, the post-season and pre-season phases are wonderful times to shift the emphasis to swimming load. For weaker swimmers who are seeking to improve their swimming (and triathlon!) performance, I often prescribe that up to 50 percent of total post-season and pre-season training hours be devoted to swimming. The benefits are a tremendous fitness foundation in swimming for the upcoming season, lower-risk training load for the musculoskeletal system, and a real opportunity to make swimming performance breakthroughs. This emphasis shift also can assist in the "shelf life" of a triathlete's emotional enjoyment and physical energy. Swimming requires frequency and load to make real improvements, and it is often impossible to do enough of this kind of work at the height of the season, when biking and running should be balanced with (or even more weighted than) swimming in your overall training load.

If running is your strength, this approach takes plenty of confidence, as you are backing off from your stronger sport for a while, but in my experience, only positive things come of it. As long as you maintain some specific positive run training, as discussed in the running chapter, and progress into a full running load throughout the rest of the season, run performance will only improve.

Setting Up Your Year

For the vast majority of the athletes I coach, I progress the swim training through four main phases of focus and emphasis. This particular setup leverages the three sports within a full-sport approach, which means that different sports will be given varying priority over the course of the season. Executed well, this setup can lead to improved fitness and recovery.

Triathlon has many types of athletes in different stages of development and with very different goals. Not every athlete would benefit from the setup discussed here. What is appropriate for an ex–elite swimmer might be very

SETTING UP WORKOUTS

Many triathletes simply hop into the pool and start swimming without any focus on progression or structure. To get the most out of your session, there is a simple and effective manner to set up all workouts. Almost every swimming session should follow this pattern.

GENERAL WARM-UP	A period of very easy swimming that prepares the body to train. Too many athletes go hard in this phase—take your time and swim very easy.
PRE–MAIN SET	We move into specificity with a set that is designed to either focus on a technical aspect, prepare you for stronger swimming in the main set, or both. This often progresses in effort and can be viewed as a bridge to the main set.
MAIN SET	This set makes up at least half of the duration of your swim workouts. By the time you begin, you should be ready to accomplish the goals of the sessions, with the "engine" fully revved up and ready to roar!
ADDITIONAL SET	You may have time to add one more short set focused on technique, open-water skills, or speed.

What you don't see here is a warm-down. I believe warm-downs to be highly overrated for triathletes, especially those with limited time. The only exception may be after very-high-intensity sessions that demand maximal exertion with high rest. Don't limit your main set to get in a warm-down!

different than what is best for an aspiring triathlete with a swimming weakness. I have made every attempt to highlight the specific areas that might warrant consideration when planning your swimming and outline a setup for the middle of the "bell curve"—that is, a good approach for triathletes who are serious about their own performance development.

Begin planning at a high level, then gradually hone the phases, weeks, and ultimately the workout progression. As I outline your season, I will first focus on a pool-swimming progression and then transition to open-water swimming. Despite the fact that you will most likely race in open water, the vast majority of your training will typically (and rightly) be completed in the pool.

Post-season Swim Training

Reduced training stress
Emphasis on technique and skills

Allow your fitness to arrive out of the frequent swim sessions, but don't chase it. Take time to focus on the technical elements, remembering not to simply "drill" to improve technique.

After the break that should occur after a season of racing, the post-season is the time to gradually rebuild some general swim conditioning while also including the greater emphasis on foundational technique work. Awareness and posture are two skills to focus on, with nearly all technique work designed to assist you in improving your alignment, posture, and tautness in the water. A great amount of work should be done with the snorkel as well as pull sets with buoy and ankle strap (and paddles for more advanced athletes). The goal in this phase is to ramp up the focus on swimming while running takes more of a backseat and to increase both the frequency of sessions and the distance swum in each session. The challenge of this phase is to swim well and prepare the body for the greater overall load that comes in the next pre-season phase.

EQUIPMENT-STRIP ENDURANCE 1

The focus in this session is to educate and execute. In other words, there is little use in working on a taut body or alignment by using pool toys if we fail to transfer those skills into proper swimming. The main set accomplishes this, all at a moderately low intensity.

Warm-up	**10 min.** easy swimming (advanced swimmers can mix strokes)
Pre–Main Set	**6 to 10 × 50** with fins (25 kick on back, 25 swim free)
	Create a taut body, with fingers and toes reaching for opposite ends of the pool.

Main Set	**3 to 4 rounds:**
	300 swim with snorkel, buoy, ankle strap at 65–70% *Working on alignment and taut body.*
	3 × 100 snorkel and ankle strap *Now working on taut body with propulsion.*
	4 × 50 swim at 80% with great form *Transferring skill to real swimming!*
Additional Set	**10 to 16 × 25**, all at 80% effort and 5 to 7 strokes per minute faster than typical cadence, with 10 sec. rest between intervals *Don't lose propulsion. This requires focus.*

SHORT-REP ENDURANCE

We aim to accomplish two things in this session. The first is to lightly build endurance without compromising form. The second is to focus on shifting alignment and proper posture into high-quality swimming. Added to this is a slightly faster stroke rate, which requires neuromuscular conditioning. We may as well start early in the season with this.

Warm-up	**300–600** very low intensity
Pre–Main Set	**6 to 8 rounds of:**
	30 sec. vertical kicking, moving to
	50 sec. swim at 80% with great form
	The focus here is to find proper posture, which is easy with vertical kicking, then maintain in swimming.
Main Set	**30 to 50 × 50** swim as
	Alternate 5 intervals with snorkel, buoy, and ankle strap, then 5 intervals at 80–85% with slightly higher stroke rate and great form; repeat until complete
	All with 10-sec. rest between intervals.
Additional Set	**10 to 16 × 25**
	Odds: 10 strokes blast fast; evens: great form at 95%

Pre-season Swim Training

Main focus is on improving cardiovascular and muscular endurance
Continued emphasis on technique and skills
Swimming may carry more emphasis than biking and running
Retain some higher-speed sessions

This is a wonderful part of the season to truly dedicate yourself to swimming development. Don't be afraid to allow the run legs to heal during this phase—they will thank you in the long run.

This is the portion of the season for establishing a firm base of fitness and muscular endurance as well as continued development of the technical aspects of swimming. For those who view swimming as their weakest leg, this part of the season often has the greatest load in swimming in terms of total weekly distance. High frequency is another key to endurance and technical improvements, often requiring a diminished focus on running during this phase. Many of the sessions are emotionally and physically challenging, although we are not aiming to make you sharp as an athlete yet—that comes closer to the primary racing season.

EQUIPMENT-STRIP ENDURANCE 2

We evolve the type of session completed in the pre-season phase to a larger main set and also place stronger emphasis on building endurance. We retain skills development in this session, despite placing equal emphasis on the heavy muscular endurance needed to properly execute the session.

Warm-up	**600** easy swimming (advanced swimmers can mix strokes)
	Remember the need to begin very light.
Pre–Main Set	**200, 175, 150, 125, 100** with snorkel, progress effort from 65% to 80%, all with 10 sec. rest
	75, 50, 25 at 80% with great form, all with 10 sec. rest
	Working on preparing the body for stronger efforts as well as proper alignment in swimming.

Main Set	**10 × 100** with snorkel, buoy, and ankle strap at 75%, with 15 sec. rest
	20 × 50 snorkel only at 80–85%, with 10 sec. rest (advanced swimmers may use paddles)
	40 × 25 swim at 85–90%, with 5 sec. rest Keep stroke rate high.
	This is a 3000-yard/meter main set. We reduce the interval length to enable you to maintain good form and proper stroke rate. Transfer posture, alignment, and propulsion into upper-endurance swimming.
Additional Set	**10 to 16 × 25** at 80% effort and 5 to 7 strokes per minute faster than typical cadence, with 10 sec. rest
	Don't lose propulsion. This requires focus.

EXTENDING INTERVAL ENDURANCE

This is a challenging, evolving main set that demands that you retain a set pace for ever-increasing distances. It ensures that you always have high awareness of the pace you are swimming as well as your pacing throughout the session. We tend to repeat this type of set every two to three weeks throughout the pre-season phase, extending the duration of the intervals.

Warm-up	**3 × 400** as 1 swim easy; 2 snorkel; 3 snorkel, buoy, ankle strap
	All easy and form-focused.
Pre–Main Set	**2 to 4 rounds:**
	200 snorkel at 70%
	3 × 50 progress 1 to 3 in effort and stroke rate to 85%
	4 × 25 fast with great form and stroke rate
	All with 10 sec. rest between intervals.
Main Set	**4 rounds with no break of:**
	100 easy at 70% with 20 sec. rest
	100 at 85% with 7–10 sec. rest (note pace and interval)
	100 easy at 70% with 20 sec. rest
	300 swim at same pace as your second 100 (85%), with 30 sec. rest Add 100 with each round—400 in round 2, 500 in 3, 600 in 4.
	This is a challenging session, but with proper pacing you will gain a big fitness yield.

Additional Set	**5 × 200** pull with snorkel, ankle strap, and buoy.
	Swim smooth and settled to find form again.

Sustained Power Swim Training

Sharpen speed and sustained power
Reduce the stress and intensity of the supporting sessions
Develop maximal sustainable speed

There is a divergence of intensity in this phase, with a reduction of intensity in the supporting and endurance sessions coupled with a heavy increase in speed in the key sessions.

Once you have established a strong foundation of muscular endurance and cardiovascular fitness, you may feel strong but not yet fast. Around the time of the spring early-season races, I like to inject a shorter phase of heavier emphasis on training that is designed to sharpen general fitness and endurance and improve your ability to hold sustained power and speed. Remember that we don't turn our backs on endurance—we still need to be selective about how often we hit maximal steady-state efforts. The key sessions of the week become sustained and very strong intervals. In spite of the fact that you may be jumping into early-season races, at this phase you will not be "race-primed." In terms of the general progression, you should have established improved technique, a strong foundation of fitness and endurance, and even improved effort at or above race pace. We have yet to get truly specific. We have yet to train for the specific demands of the event!

BEST SUSTAINED EFFORT 100S

This session requires high effort and proper pacing, and it is too easy to be a "passenger" here while failing to truly give your best effort. While it doesn't look overly daunting, this one hurts. You must be prepared to swim fast by the main set.

Warm-up	**500** easy swimming (advanced swimmers can mix strokes)
	Remember the need to begin very light.
Pre–Main Set 1	Pull with snorkel, buoy, and ankle strap:
	2 × 200 at 70%
	2 × 150 at 75%
	2 × 100 at 80%
	2 × 50 at 85%
Pre–Main Set 2	**20 × 25** as 5 rounds of 4 x 25 progressing each interval as easy, build, fast, faster (advanced swimmers may use paddles)
	Hit top-end speed.
Main Set	**4 to 6 rounds:**
	4 × 100 at your best sustained effort with 30 sec. rest
	4 × 100 at 60% with buoy with 15 sec. rest
	Rest 90 sec. between rounds.
Additional Set	**800** pull smooth with choice of equipment and great form

PROGRESSIVE INTENSITY

While the focus is top-end speed, I like to set athletes up for success, especially when I consider that we are managing three disciplines in triathlon. Progressive efforts allow athletes to feel good and retain great form and often result in the highest-quality sessions. In addition, there are big pacing lessons within these types of sessions.

Warm-up	**10 min.** very easy swimming
Pre–Main Set	**1500** pull with snorkel, buoy, and ankle strap, swim as:
	200, 100, 2 × 150, 2 × 75, 3 × 100, 3 × 50, 4 × 50, 4 × 25, progressing effort from 65% to 85% throughout the set
	All with 10 sec. rest between intervals.

Main Set	**6 × 250** with 45 sec. rest Progress speed and effort as: 1 at 80%, 2 at 85–90%, 3 at best effort; repeat progression
	300 with buoy at 70% with 30 sec. rest
	6 × 200 with 45 sec. rest Progress speed and effort as: 1 at 80%, 2 at 85–90%, 3 at best effort; repeat progression
	300 with buoy at 70% with 30 sec. rest
	6 × 150 with 45 sec. rest Progress speed and effort as: 1 at 80%, 2 at 85–90%, 3 at best effort; repeat progression
	300 with buoy at 70% with 30 sec. rest
	6 × 100 with 45 sec. rest Progress speed and effort as: 1 at 80%, 2 at 85–90%, 3 at best effort; repeat progression
	Notice how the rest remains despite the duration of the interval decreasing!
Additional Set	**5 rounds** with paddles:
	50 easy with 20 sec. rest
	2 × 25 fast, keep stroke rate up, with 15 sec. rest
	Then done.

Race-Specific Swim Training

Retain similar focus for all distances of racing for your preparation
Mimic race-specific skills and familiarity
Manipulate interval distance to match your event focus

Many triathletes are fearful of the swim, but much of this fear comes from a lack of familiarity. If you can simulate the sensations and experiences of the race scenario, you will arrive both fit and confident. That is the key to maximize speed and also to reduce emotional stress and cost.

The longest phase of the training year covers the bulk of the racing season, and the entire focus is to train for the experience, demands, and skills of open-water racing. This includes open-water-specific skills, race simulators, and sessions to get you highly familiar with the sensations and feelings that accompany racing.

It's my hope that you will make specific skills, such as sighting, such a habit that they will require no thought and won't inhibit speed during the race. We also want to train to make the highly uncomfortable experiences, such as take-out effort, transitions out of the water, or close contact with other athletes, so familiar that they don't lead to panic or take up emotional energy. This familiarity will free you to focus on effort, navigation, and tactics, or, as we like to call it, the ability to *impose yourself on the race.*

OPEN-WATER SESSION

Pool swimming is a wonderful way to build fitness, work on form, and complete the majority of your training, but it lacks the specificity of the dynamic environment of open-water swimming. Properly designed open-water sessions are the only way to truly prepare for open-water racing. You will note the value of small-group training in this session.

Warm-up	**10 min.** easy swimming to get used to the environment
Pre–Main Set	**5 × 1 min.,** progress effort from 1 to 5 to 85% with 30 sec. rest
Main Set	*Choose a loop with beach start and finish and buoy turns, if possible.* **3 to 4 rounds** of a loop (4–6 min.): Loop 1: 75–80% with sighting every sixth stroke: work on skills Loop 2: First and last 100 strokes fast with sighting, middle of swim at 80% Loop 3: Full race-simulation effort (fast!) with proper sighting, navigation, and beach start/finish All with 1 min. rest between intervals.

POOL RACE-SIMULATION SESSION

We can mimic the feeling and stress of open-water racing in a pool. You will be amazed at the race adaptation and familiarity that occur following a few of these types of sessions. Please note the skills integration in the pre–main set. We are always working on race-specific skills now.

Warm-up	10 min. easy swimming with mix of strokes
Pre–Main Set 1	**4 × 400** swim each 400 as: 50 easy 50 with 10 strokes faster stroke rate 50 with 15 strokes faster stroke rate 50 with 20 strokes faster stroke rate Always sighting every sixth stroke throughout the swim. Rest 1 min between sets. Repeat progression.
Pre–Main Set 2	**9 to 12 × 50** progress effort from 1 to 3 to fast (90%), all with higher stroke rate, with 20 sec. rest between intervals
Main Set	**3 to 5 rounds:** **3 to 4 × 50** at 90% effort, with 20 sec. rest All are with a deck-up and dive (hop out of pool once you touch, stand, turn, and prepare to dive in for the coming interval) *This greatly elevates breathing and heart rate and puts swimmers under duress, like a race start.* **300–600** at race-specific intensity, sighting every sixth stroke **6 × 25** easy recovery between rounds

MAXIMAL SUSTAINED EFFORT

We always want to maintain your maximal sustained effort throughout the race-specific phase, as this top-end work will retain the top-end swimming ability. It is easy to retain some focus on race-specific skills development even in a session such as this.

Warm-up	**300** loose and very easy
Pre–Main Set	**12 × 100** as: 1–4 with snorkel, buoy, and ankle strap at 70% 5–8 100s with paddles and ankle strap at 80% 9–12 100s swim with great form at 85% **800** progress effort by 200 with sighting every sixth stroke throughout

Main Set	**3 × 200** progress effort to close to best effort (95%), with 45 sec. rest
	200s swim at that same pace with 1 min. rest.
	Once you fail to maintain the pace (±2 sec.) at the 200 distance, **drop your interval distance to 150** with 1 min. rest.
	Once you fail to maintain that pace (±2 sec.) at the 150 distance, **drop your interval distance to 100** with 1 min rest.
	Do no more than 12 swims, including the initial 3 × 200.

7

Cycling in Triathlon

Bike for show and run for dough" is an old saying commonly heard in triathlon circles. The implication is that many athletes ride strong and keen to impress but that real performance arrives out of a solid run. There is an element of truth to this idea because a good run is essential to a great overall performance, but this sentiment devalues the importance of a well-executed bike ride. The bike portion of the race typically requires the most time to complete, often up to 50 percent of the total race time, yet cycling remains the triathlon discipline that many athletes take for granted.

The grand middle discipline of triathlon carries the same importance as the other disciplines. Not only does cycling have much potential for real time gains, it will also greatly influence your run performance. Your level of effort and exertion will decide how much your ride "costs" you, which is why a great deal of physical and emotional focus should be placed on your riding training. In this chapter I will outline where the riding leg fits within your sport and explain how to become a better rider. A sound approach to cycling opens many doors of opportunity to improve and refine both efficiency and speed.

Many triathletes think of swimming as the most technical of the three sports, but performance cycling involves many technical decisions. Unlike swimming and running, cycling requires a significant piece of equipment—

the bicycle. After you select a bike, several details require special attention and consideration: how you sit on your bike, how you interact with it, and how you manage your effort. Once you understand how these aspects of your riding help or hinder your speed and energy cost, the route to improvement becomes clear. If you focus only on the skills of balance and pedaling and then rely on the basic intervals and rides associated with training as the simple sources for all improvements, you will probably be disappointed! If you truly wish to evolve your riding performance and, in turn, facilitate improved running off the bike, you'll need to spend some time working on the technical aspects of cycling.

Rather than diving into the minutiae of bike fit or merely outlining the intervals or training schedule that will improve your riding, I will outline a vision of how you should view your riding training and all that it encompasses. Here's my logic: Before you consider what types of riding and intervals will provide improvements, you must first be aware of *how to ride the bike well*. In the longer term, riding the bike well is the route to real and lasting change, and it will provide a platform for massive performance gains. Before we delve into this, let's investigate the traditional approach to triathlon riding and dispel some of the harmful myths that inhibit improvements.

DEBUNKING THE MYTHS OF TRIATHLON CYCLING

If you step back to observe the bike training practiced by most athletes and recommended by most coaches, or read the headlines in triathlon media, you will see that everyone seems to talk about better performance being the result of a focused approach to accumulating miles (or hours) on the bicycle and improving on commercially driven components of the bike and its setup—bike fit and power meters. Granted, time on the bicycle is a critical part of becoming an improved rider, a proper bike fit is key to success, and power meters are great tools for training and racing. The problem is that too many athletes and coaches are lulled into focusing only on these areas, and they don't move the conversation further.

MYTH: **Training volume is directly correlated with training response.** For many athletes the number of miles ridden in a day or week is the primary indicator of a job well done—80 miles is 80 miles, and time on the seat surely equals success. If only this were true! Unfortunately, most of riders do not spend much, if any, time really thinking about *how* these miles are ridden or *how effectively* they actually ride their bikes.

The focus on volume is compounded by a lack of training progression and specificity. Most triathletes execute a training plan that calls for a narrow range of intensity throughout each ride and over the course of a week of training. Their narrow bandwidth for intensity is complemented by an equally narrow range of cadences deployed at any part of a bike ride. Fluctuations happen only when the terrain forces them. In order to become a better triathlete, you must adopt a progressive training focus on the bike.

MYTH: **Focus on power to improve performance.** Loiter in any triathlon forum or eavesdrop on the pre-race chat between competitors, and you will hear plenty of discussion about average power, functional threshold, and heart rate as measures of riding performance. The common goal is to set up the bicycle in an optimal fashion, then train to "hold a specific power output" for the duration of the race. There's no denying that power can provide great gains when taken in context, but there is little consideration of how an athlete should plan to deploy his or her available power (or work) on different terrains, in variable conditions, and on different courses.

MYTH: **Bike fit is everything.** The pursuit of the most aero position is important for triathletes, but there's a caveat: Look for the most aerodynamic position on the bike that still allows you to maintain good posture and proper pedaling mechanics. These are absolutely critical components of bike and rider setup, and for most triathletes the process will be an ongoing one.

MYTH: **Triathlon is a constant steady-state event.** Triathlon racing is viewed as demanding a steady and sustained effort within a very narrow range of power or effort. While it certainly has steady-state characteristics compared with sports such as road cycling, you will not deliver your most effective bike leg and set up a high-quality run by holding heart rate and power perfectly steady unless you are on a flat and completely windless bike course. You must achieve balance between cardiovascular and muscular stress, and it is possible to shift between them. This point takes us into training for triathlon: You must train to develop different tools that can then be utilized in different terrains and parts of the race to ensure that your effort is productive, not destructive!

MYTH: **Long, slow distance is king.** Training in a single band on the lower end of the intensity spectrum will only prevent you from reaching your riding potential. To truly evolve as a rider, you need a healthy diet of lower-intensity training, however, you want to touch every intensity available within any given week of training. The key is to dose the intensity prescription and ratio relative to where you are at in the season. You'll find much more on this in the training section of the chapter.

MYTH: **Junk miles are OK.** In my mind, there is no place for junk miles in triathlon training. Low-intensity, easy miles have great value, but only if you are engaged and thinking about your riding. Every mile should have a purpose, and low-intensity miles provide the opportunity for you to work on posture, gear selection, pedal stroke, and other highly valuable elements of awareness and skill. Make it your goal for posture, handling skills, and gear selection to become so habitual that they require little to no thought. If you are successful, you will be able to put more willpower and thought into managing your effort and riding varied terrain.

MYTH: **Moving your position farther forward is better.** In the sport of triathlon we are able to set up a rider in a very forward position relative to the bottom bracket. This position allows us to open up the hip angle without having to perch on the tip of the saddle (which many road time trialists will do to conform to regulations). This doesn't mean that moving forward from your current position will be optimal. Pushing your position too far forward will compromise the power you can generate because it limits the range and time you have to recruit the muscles in the back of the leg.

MYTH: **Getting out of the saddle is a waste of energy.** I see many athletes religiously sit in their time trial bars throughout the entire race, often not to their benefit. It can be very efficient to remain in an aero position for large portions of racing, but there are several situations when it is advantageous to come out of the saddle and add body weight to efficient pedaling to regain, maintain, or increase momentum. Standing also relieves the postural stress or load that results from extended periods spent in the time trial position.

BENEFITS OF IMPROVED CYCLING

Triathlon performance is fundamentally about maximizing speed while managing energy usage. In longer events, such as Ironman-distance or half-Ironman-distance races, improved riding resilience and performance not only improve your splits but can also save critical energy that allows your running potential to blossom. The most obvious example is Olympic-distance racing, especially draft-legal races, in which the constant and rapidly changing tactical situation further emphasizes the need to minimize stress by being a competent and confident bike rider.

I encourage you to view cycling as the bedrock of your triathlon potential because it can lead to the following advantages:

Time gains. The potential for faster bike splits is an obvious advantage. At the end of the day, whether you aim to win a world championship or simply improve your best performance, going faster is always desirable.

Reduced energy cost. Becoming a stronger cyclist opens up the potential to be in greater control of your energy deployment throughout the cycling portion of the race. In turn, this opens up opportunities for you to minimize cost while maximizing speed.

Improved run performance. You can never truly maximize run performance and overall triathlon performance if you haven't fully developed your riding ability. You will be forced to ride conservatively in order to run well off the bike. Even if your run performance appears solid, you are making sacrifices in terms of your overall performance.

Master your interaction with the bike, the terrain, and the course, and you will perform better both on the run and in the overall race.

AN INTRODUCTION TO RIDING AWARENESS

In getting started, I want you to focus on learning how to ride your bike. If your competition is piling on miles and focusing on fit and power, this presents a real opportunity for you! It doesn't matter what type of intervals you do, how many miles you accumulate, or how aerodynamic your position is if you don't understand the three levels of riding awareness and train to improve them. It's the only way to get closer to your riding, or triathlon, performance potential. By immersing yourself in the project of becoming a better rider you will maximize your speed in relation to the energy and effort expended. The speed you gain is "purchased" with emotional investment during training—there is no such thing as "free speed."

We must consider the bigger picture before we dive into specific skills and preparation. The physiological preparation required to improve cycling places a heavy emphasis on progression and specificity. The same approach can be applied to developing this riding awareness. In the early part of seasonal training, there is generally less focus on stressful intervals, allowing a greater capacity for the emotional focus that skills and handling require. Focusing on this type of training early in the season will make good riding form more habitual, leaving greater capacity for stressful intervals later in the season. By the time you are ready to race, you might need to check "form before force" periodically, but your mental energy will largely be free to apply good riding form to the course, including making the best use of terrain, managing hydration and nutrition, and even beginning to prepare for the run toward the end of the ride.

Good form becomes critical when racing the back half of a ride, when triathletes typically experience a gradual decline in physical resources. This is both natural and inevitable if you are riding close to your potential. If your riding form is underdeveloped, the decline of your physical resources will be multiplied by a decline in form. Nowhere is this more important than in races such as the Hawaii Ironman, where you may earn considerable time gains over your competition in the last 30 miles of the ride. In the 2009 Ironman World Championships, Chris Lieto, who is known to be a skilled cyclist, gained almost 9 minutes over the final 25 miles of the bike course without altering his power output. While this gain marked his ability to impose himself on his competition, it also illustrates how declining form and energy made for a sharp drop-off in performance for others leading the pack.

We will attack the three levels of awareness in riding performance in order of priority. Until you master level one, you cannot effectively focus on and improve level two, and unless the first two are refined, the third is irrelevant. In this chapter we will discuss two essential elements of triathlon riding:

- Mastering how you interact with your bicycle
- Mastering how you interact with the terrain and course

After mastering these two elements of riding, you can turn your attention to how you impose yourself on others during the race. I hasten to add that many of the elite athletes whom I coach are still working on the first two elements of riding. While these elements of riding are usually an afterthought, they are critical to unlocking your riding potential.

LEVEL 1 | Interaction with Your Bike

There are several considerations that have a great impact on how effectively you ride your bike: equipment and position, postural awareness, pedal stroke, and riding skills. Of course better riding skills can only be developed by riding outside, but the other components can be worked on in a controlled environment, indoors on a trainer. Better position, postural fitness, and a more efficient pedal stroke will set the stage for better riding skills, so let's begin there.

Optimizing Position

The goal of a proper triathlon bike fit is to find a *sustainable* aerodynamic position that allows you to maintain good pedaling for extended periods and bring maximal resources to the final effort of the race: running. Being as aerodynamic as possible is not advantageous if you cannot sustain good form in that position. Keep this in mind if you opt to work with professional bike fitters. They are a valuable resource as long as they embrace the practical aspect of a sustainable fit. Keep in mind that all fit issues can not be solved in a single trainer-based session.

Moving into a more aerodynamic position creates a few fit-related issues due to the fact that your riding position moves horizontally in relation to the ground (Figure 7.1). Stay with me as I dive into a little technical explanation. The shortest distance from the bottom bracket to the top of your saddle is a vertical line, and most triathletes sit behind this line. (Note that the bottom bracket is the center of the rotation of the cranks.) As your point of contact with the saddle moves forward toward this line, the change effectively lowers your seat. Conversely, if you position yourself farther behind this line, your seat is effectively higher.

The farther forward you move, the shorter your range of engagement will be for the large muscles on the back of the leg, including the hamstrings. Due to the effect of both gravity and pelvic structure, there will come a point where you are unable to rotate further.

FIGURE 7.1 ¦ POSITION IN RELATION TO BOTTOM BRACKET

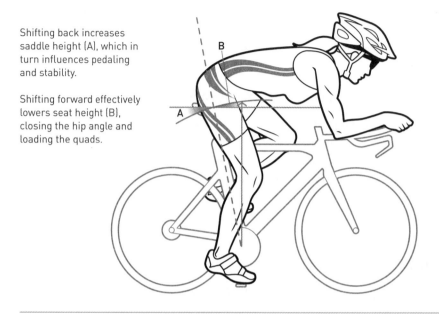

Shifting back increases saddle height (A), which in turn influences pedaling and stability.

Shifting forward effectively lowers seat height (B), closing the hip angle and loading the quads.

Changing your posture on the bike produces alterations in "real position." Awareness of these compromises will minimize their effects but also highlights the benefit of finding a sustainable aerodynamic position and maintaining a focus on good posture.

Why is this relevant to triathlon bike fit? Let's assume that your fit was completed in your most comfortable and sustainable aero position while in a heavier gear, so as to achieve an accurate leg length. When you go for a ride, you find you have the tendency to move forward on the saddle from your original fitted position, which effectively lowers your seat height and potentially places a significant load on your legs. While climbing, you find that you move back on the saddle, a very common practice. In the climbing position you find yourself reaching for the pedals because you have effectively created an elevated seat height by sitting farther behind that vertical line that extends from your bottom bracket. Interestingly, this effect is magnified when you sit up out of the time trial position and still further magnified by the stepped design of some popular triathlon-specific saddles. All this goes to illustrate that simply getting fitted in a lab does not assure a proper position throughout your riding on the road.

Five Considerations for a Proper Triathlon Fit

The touchpoints of bike equipment are your shoes, saddle, shorts, and bars. Choose the most effective and practical options within your budget. Once you have a bike that is the correct size for you, it becomes a process of fitting and testing to find the optimal position for you. Remember: *Getting the fit points right is a positive step, but being able to hold posture on the bike is paramount.*

1. Seat Choice

A proper fit on the right saddle will allow you to maximize power and efficiency and hold a stable position in the saddle. It's a highly individual choice, so don't be swayed by other athletes' opinions or by product reviews. Being uncomfortable in the saddle leads to a subconscious backward rotation of the pelvis. This shift changes your fit, leads to a loss of power and efficiency, and causes too much movement on the bike (less propulsion).

Put the most comfortable, supportive part of your saddle under your most efficient position—there's no reason to perch on the tip of your saddle.

If you find yourself wanting to tilt the front of the saddle down to solve the comfort problem, you are merely treating a symptom. The cause of your discomfort could be inappropriate saddle selection, fit (for example, the seat is not under you or your setup is too long), or posture. Furthermore, when you tilt the front of the saddle down, it creates stress in the upper body because you are constantly pushing back to counter the effects of gravity and pedaling that make you slide forward.

2. Cranks

Crank length can significantly impact your position on the bike. Switching to shorter cranks will allow you to sustain a more aerodynamic position and achieve a more open hip angle (the angle between the thigh and torso). In aero position, your knees will not be as close to your chest at the top of the pedal stroke, which means you can increase comfort and/or efficiency, lower your position for improved aerodynamics, or get a bit of all three. Being more aerodynamic has a big impact on speed, and sparing energy and postural stress means you will be in a better place coming off the bike and into the run. Longer cranks can lead to a setup where the hip angle is tighter, which in turn impedes the athlete's ability to find good posture and running biomechanics once the run starts. (For more on cranks, see "Use Shorter Cranks to Your Advantage," page 151.)

Shifting to shorter cranks is not a cure-all for improved riding performance and running off the bike, but the feedback from pros through amateurs has been overwhelmingly positive. Furthermore, it seems to require little to no time to adapt to the shorter cranks, meaning this is a risk-free alteration to your setup, with no learning curve.

3. Aero Bar Setup

You will spend about 90 percent of your time in an aero position so it is important that the position be comfortable, sustainable, and sufficiently aerodynamic. Believe it or not, these things are not mutually exclusive. There are a number of helpful guides for establishing the range of workable angles for upper-body aero fit, which will allow you to appropriately position the armrests under your elbows and torso. Less attention has been given to establishing usable space between the hip and shoulder to allow a flat or consistently gentle curve to the back that opens up the diaphragm. It becomes possible to achieve a relatively flat aero position without a large drop to the pads if you think about the setup in this way.

Pad width and height also need to take breathing into account. Extension length and bend should allow for an intuitive and relaxed wrist position and ease of use for shifting and should include a comfortable position cue such as thumb on top or finger wrapped around shifter. While straight extensions look cool when your bike is parked outside the café, if they compromise long-distance comfort, your performance will suffer.

4. Secondary Controls

Little attention is paid to the position of the bullhorns, yet their placement is critical if you are to develop the various necessary non-aero interactions with your bike. It is common to see bikes set up with base bars too low and/or too close to the rider. This is one of the challenges in choosing and setting up some of the new integrated superbike front ends. As a rough guide, aim for bullhorn reach and height in the range that would fall between just below well-positioned brake hoods and drops on a road bike. If your triathlon bike is your only bike, pay attention to this aspect of setup to vastly increase the day-to-day usability of your bike.

One of the most significant improvements in tri bike equipment is electronic shifting from the bullhorn position, which facilitates more intuitive interactions with the bike.

TRI FITTING ON A ROAD BIKE

Many newer triathletes or recreational triathletes utilize a road bike fitted with clip-on bars to create a time trial bike. There is nothing wrong with this approach, but it has limitations. Attaining a long-distance tri fit on a road bike can be difficult due to the geometric differences between road and time trial or tri-specific bikes—front/rear center dimensions, seat and head tube angles, and weight distribution. Bike handling and steering can be compromised if the rider is positioned as far forward as a tri bike to lower the aero profile and open up the hip angle.

5. Shorts, Pedals, and Shoes

Much time and effort can go into a bike fit only for it to be corrupted by the simple fact of training in a comfortable thickly padded cycling short and racing in a thinly padded tri short. The variance in shape and thickness can change your effective saddle height and often causes a different forward-aft orientation. It is not uncommon for athletes to blame the saddle for issues that are caused by their cycling shorts. To address this problem, find a comfortable race short option and get several pairs. Then optimize your bike setup wearing your race shorts, and when you swap shorts, be aware of the compromises that result.

A similar situation exists with shoes—be aware of differences in sole thickness and cleat forward/aft position. The position of the shoe cleat is the point where the whole bike position originates, and its orientation is critical to ensure good pedaling alignment and injury prevention. (Note that not all pedal systems suit all pedaling styles and biomechanics.)

Don't worry about achieving perfect symmetry in your fit with regard to foot orientation. We start asymmetrical, and over time learned behaviors further contribute to asymmetry. There are some useful fitting tools to help avoid injury; however, in adult athletes, attempting to force symmetry often leads to problems elsewhere.

One final note on bike fit for triathletes: Triathlon is not restricted by the UCI (International Cycling Federation) rules on position that road cyclists face. Consequently, as much can be discarded as learned from studying road time trialists' positions.

Choosing Your Equipment

Regardless of how high up the tri-bike-shopping tree you choose to climb, there are some basic ideas worth considering. The latest, greatest superbikes will arrive with much fanfare, but nothing in life comes without compromise. Sleek, aerodynamic designs often compromise ease of use in daily life. Please don't be fooled into purchasing anything simply because it's more aerodynamic. Remember that your position on the bike is the primary factor affecting performance for both propulsion and up to 75 percent of aero drag (wheels, frame, and accessories make up the balance). Don't get me wrong—faster equipment is good, but it is more important to pull a reliable, cleanly built bike from the rack on race day, knowing it fits well and is enjoyable to ride.

Learn how to clean your bike, assemble it, and check that it is functioning correctly. Don't leave home without knowing how to change a flat in a timely, stress-free manner. Always carry equipment-specific spares and tools, and know how to use your tire inflator. You have not prepared properly for your race if you have not practiced this aspect of the sport, and the practice will be useful should you find yourself under duress on race day.

Know how to measure the key points of contact on your bike and record them. It's helpful to have a reference if adjustments need to be made later.

Crank Length

If you are riding a triathlon bike with longer cranks, thinking it will give you more leverage and thus higher power output, you should reconsider. Remember that our goal is to ride as fast as we can, then run well off the bike. There's more to the equation than simply maximal pedal force, especially if it comes at the cost of aerodynamics, comfort, run performance, and so on. Shorter cranks offer triathletes tangible benefits with few or no compromises.

Wheels

With today's modern wheels, it is perfectly acceptable to use just one set of wheels for both training and racing. If you choose to do this, it is worth keeping a set of tires for training, then switching to a different set of race tires to reduce the risk of race-day flats. If you have more than one set of wheels, consider the following issues:

- Freehub body/cassette spacing can be slightly different from one brand to the next, which will alter gear tuning.

USE SHORTER CRANKS TO YOUR ADVANTAGE

Crank length is measured from the center of the bottom bracket to the center of the pedal spindle. The diagram below compares the difference between a typical long crank (172.5 mm) and a shorter crank (165 mm) to show the advantage of using shorter cranks.

- Shorter cranks effectively shorten the distance to the bottom of the pedal stroke, 6 o'clock (A), and the distance to the top of the pedal stroke, 12 o'clock (B).

- The reach to the bottom of the pedal stroke, or the 6 o'clock position, is driven by the individual rider's physiology (e.g., height, femur length, flexibility), so it remains constant regardless of the crank length. The diagram shows that the reach for both long and short cranks is the same.

- Because reach is constant, the shorter cranks require that the seat be raised to adjust for the difference in crank length (C is higher to keep R1 constant).

- The shorter cranks create 15 mm of additional space compared with the longer cranks. The diagram shows that X2 is longer than X1. This extra space enables a more open hip angle (the angle created between torso and femur).

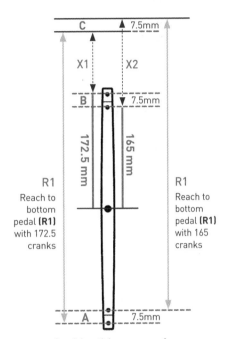

Crank length is a measure from the center of the bottom bracket to center of pedal spindle.

- The knee does not have to rise as high to reach the top of the pedal stroke, so the position is less scrunched. In aero position, when the foot is at the top of the pedal stroke, there will be more distance between the knee and the chest. This has the potential to positively affect aerodynamics, efficiency, and comfort.

- Brake track height and width may vary and require resetting brakes for proper operation.
- Deeper isn't always better—consider crosswind performance.

Tires

- Balance advertised speed with reliability—most really light race tires get to be that way through less rubber and reduced puncture protection.
- Inflation pressure is critical to performance speed and grip.
- Check your tires for embedded debris prior to racking your bike.
- Ensure that the valve stem is long enough to fit the Pit Stop canister, if that's what you plan to use.

Gearing

- Keep in mind that the fresh cassette on your race wheels might not interact well with the tired chain on your bike.
- Choose gear ratios that are broad enough to deal with the course's features.
- For flatter courses, close ratio (11/23) will mean smaller jumps between gears, which makes it easier to be in just the right gear.
- If resources permit, consider smaller or larger front chainring options for climbing courses or those with long, gradual descents.
- Electronic shifting incorporating a base-bar option is one of the best advances in tri bike equipment because it allows easier application of different riding tools and more fluid progress over challenging terrain. If your tri bike is your only bike, base-bar shifting greatly improves its day-to-day usability.

Developing Postural Fitness

Being able to sit on your bike in a controlled and relaxed way is one of the cornerstones to improved performance. Good posture is not only essential for efficiency and good riding form but is also a key component to handling your bike in a fluid, intuitive way. We can and should practice good posture every time we interact with the bike, indoors or out. Because it eliminates the distractions of the environment, the indoor trainer is the perfect place to work on this most basic and important aspect of performance, as is your road bike if you have one.

FIGURE 7.2 | **POSTURAL FITNESS IN AERO POSITION**

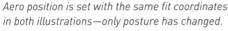

*Aero position is set with the same fit coordinates
in both illustrations—only posture has changed.*

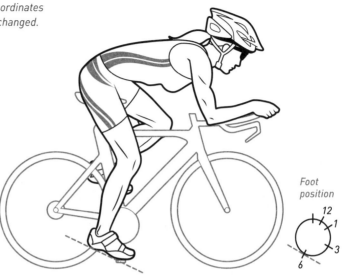

GOOD POSTURE

The athlete's pelvis is rotated
forward, the back is flat, and the
upper body remains relaxed; the
diaphragm is not stressed. The
hands are forward on the time
trial bar extenders. Good posture
improves power and economy as
a result of a more open hip angle
and a sound aero position.

*Foot
position*

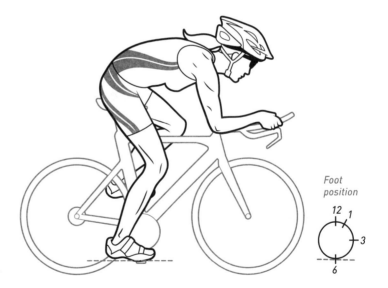

POOR POSTURE

Despite a good fit, the rider's
pelvis is rotated backward,
causing the back to be hunched
and the athlete to "choke back"
on the aerobars, holding tension
in the shoulders. Poor posture
reduces power and economy,
places additional load on the
body, and makes it difficult for
the athlete to run well off the bike.

*Foot
position*

Note on foot position: *Many triathletes have a tendency to tip the toes down at the bottom of the pedal stroke when
riding in aero position. The angle of the foot is often relative to the rotation of the pelvis. The entire "clock face of
pedaling" rotates forward with the pelvis, tipping the clock and increasing the foot angle. This is yet another reason
not to overthink ankle position in pedaling.*

FIGURE 7.3 | POSTURAL FITNESS COMING OUT OF TIME TRIAL POSITION

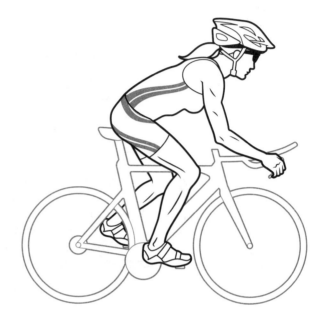

GOOD POSTURE

The athlete's pelvis is rotated forward, the back is flat, and the upper body remains relaxed; the diaphragm is not stressed. The hands are forward on the time trial bar extenders. Good posture improves power and economy as a result of a more open hip angle and a sound aero position.

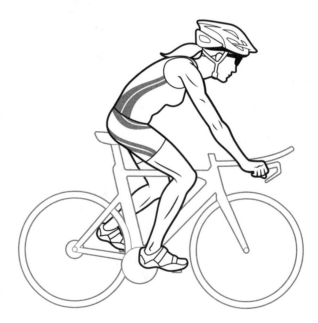

POOR POSTURE

Despite a good fit, the rider's pelvis is rotated backward, causing the back to be hunched and the athlete to "choke back" on the aerobars, holding tension in the shoulders. Poor posture reduces power and economy, places additional load on the body, and makes it difficult for the athlete to run well off the bike.

PRACTICING POSTURAL FITNESS

Most athletes have the core strength to ride with good posture; what is required is neuromuscular awareness. Try this on the indoor trainer: Sit up vertically with your arms dangling at your sides while pedaling slowly in a heavy gear. Lean forward slowly from the waist and feel the muscles in the lower back engage. Just before you topple forward, drape your hands over the base bar. Those muscles in the lower back that your brain is now talking to aid in stabilizing the pelvis when you are pushing hard on the pedals. We have all stood up and hyperextended the back on a long climb to relieve these muscles, only to sit down and think, "Wow, my legs feel better." The legs don't get stronger, but their effort now goes down through the drivetrain rather than being dissipated through the upper body. By working on your postural fitness, not only will you look good but you will also ride easier and go faster.

Postural fitness is especially important in Ironman racing—it is very difficult to stand tall while running if you have just spent many hours folded up on the bike with only a small distance between your shoulders and hips. There are some wonderful tools, including computer programs, that can help set up an optimal fit, but don't neglect the human element of the equation. Without ongoing assessment and adequate fitness to maintain good posture for the duration of your riding, the fit becomes close to worthless.

Postural fitness is developed through riding experience, good musculoskeletal integrity, improved mobility, and awareness of how you are holding your body on the bike. The best bike fit can be destroyed by "lying" on the bike incorrectly. In Figures 7.2 and 7.3, the touchpoints of the fit are the same in both illustrations; we simply altered how the rider is holding herself. Awareness and postural fitness are key to bike riding (and running and swimming!).

The Pedal Stroke

The goal of pedaling is to maintain tension on the chain throughout the pedal stroke to maximize the speed of your bike. A good pedal stroke actually begins "upstairs." There is little to no gain from movement or tension in the upper body when you are pedaling. If you are maintaining good posture, you should be able to keep a good distance between shoulders and hips, allowing free breathing. A supple and open upper body is the foundation of pedaling. Now we move "downstairs" to focus on power production—the legs!

Cues for Postural Fitness & Effective Pedaling

- Fingers relaxed
- Wrists straight in both planes
- Elbows flexed downward
- Neck and shoulders relaxed
- Controlled breathing and heart rate
- Sitting in the correct part of the saddle
- Recovering the foot through the bottom of the stroke
- Unweighting the retreating foot
- Relaxing the foot

Imagine your pedal stroke as a clock face (looking at the bike from the drive side). You simply cannot create even force around the entire pedal stroke. Much of the power generated on the bike is the result of the force applied between 1 and 5 o'clock on the clock face. This will never change, as it is where your biomechanical setup is optimized for force production. Your pedal stroke is similar to many other athletic activities, such as rowing, which relies on specific muscle sequencing to allow load to be transferred with maximum biomechanical advantage from one working muscle group to the next group before the first has reached the end of its useful range. In cycling, the powerful downstroke occurs between 1 and 5 o'clock, but a transition of sequencing needs to be initiated by the time your driving leg is at 4 o'clock. This process links your pedal strokes together to ensure a fluid application of force. Eliminating the negative force of a lazy retreating leg between 7 and 11 o'clock is the next focus. Finally we minimize the least biomechanically efficient part of the stroke, from 11 to 1 o'clock. Still with me?

If we put a child on a bicycle, they will push down on the pedals and accelerate. The push-down phase between 1 and 5 o'clock is instinctive and utilizes the powerful quadriceps muscles, which requires little neuromuscular training. Unfortunately, if we just push down, the rolling resistance, wind resistance, and gravity will slow the bike down between pedal strokes. To improve speed and riding effectiveness, we must train the counterintuitive part of the pedal stroke, in which the muscles in the back of the leg are used to link one downstroke with the other. The result? Constant tension on the chain and the most speed relative to effort. We go faster in a more effective manner.

As we discuss the pedal stroke, it is important to mention "ankling." Your most efficient pedal stroke is the result of applying force in a circular fashion, always perpendicular to the crank arm. As long as this is achieved, it makes very little difference whether you have a pronounced fluid flexion of the ankle or a relatively rigid ankle. Athletes are often taught to overexaggerate the ankling motion, but seldom with any positive results. In general terms, higher cadences often result in the toe being more pointed and heel up, while at higher loads and lower cadences, the heel is lower through the bottom of the stroke. If you isolate the different pedaling quadrants and are aware of the circular path of your foot, the ankle will sort itself out. The ankle is not, for the typical athlete, something that requires real thought.

 TIP *Be aware that "clawing" with the toes through the bottom of the stroke introduces unnecessary stress in the lower leg. It's a problem that can often be cured by simple awareness, but it is sometimes linked to shoe-fit issues.*

A final note to consider in refining your pedal stroke is symmetry of your right and left legs. Almost every rider has a more dominant leg in his or her pedal stroke. This is entirely normal. Whether asymmetry is a learned behavior or the result of compensation following injury, the dominant leg works harder through the bottom of the pedal stroke and the heel drops between 5 and 7 o'clock. The losses as a result of asymmetry are modest, but a more balanced pedal stroke makes it easier to run well off the bike. Single-leg drills on the trainer allow us to isolate each leg and reprogram the brain to "talk to" the muscles in sequence. Done in isolation, the drills can prevent any distraction and improve recruitment and power potential for the weaker leg. Of course,

---

PRACTICING PEDAL STROKE WITH SINGLE-LEG DRILLS

- Following a proper warm-up, unclip one foot and pedal at a cadence of 40–60 rpm. The slower cadence will give you time to think through each quadrant of the pedal stroke.
- Begin with 1-min. intervals with each leg, followed by 1 min. of regular riding (with both legs) between intervals.
- Progress the intervals to multiple sets of up to 3 min. on each leg.
- It's a good idea to complete one extra set on your weak leg to integrate this skills-based session.

---

you don't have to be on a trainer to focus on good pedaling form. Simply *focus* on one leg at a time, one quadrant at a time, throughout a ride. Truly focusing on a leg and thinking about each part of the stroke throughout a ride makes for a massive neuromuscular stimulus.

Riding Skills

To evolve your triathlon riding, you must place heavy focus and attention on improving your bike-handling skills to become an efficient and effective rider. These are the skills we can improve only while riding outside. Of course, a good fit and ability to maintain posture are important factors, but the ultimate goal is to eliminate any inefficient, destructive, or counterproductive aspects of riding, hence gaining speed or energy with less accumulated stress. I want you to think about how you are riding your bike instead of simply riding.

Consider whether you spend much, or any, time truly focusing on these riding skills. The following list is not a comprehensive one, but it will begin to open the door to improved riding skills.

Use of Gears

The gearing on your bike is there to allow you to choose the load and cadence over varying terrain and conditions. Appropriate smooth gear selection is a basic riding skill that, when executed poorly, results in sudden under- or overgearing and a loss of momentum. Become more familiar with the relationship and crossover between your big and small front chainrings and your rear cassette. Practice shifting fluidly between them on different gradients. For example, if you are using 53×39 front rings on a constant uphill gradient, you will generally select two harder gears at the rear as you drop from the big to small ring to arrive in the next easiest gear. Learn to plan your shifts. Look up at the gradient ahead, and if you are going to be consistently below 18 mph, shift to the small ring.

Braking

Good braking protocol generally involves progressive and even applications of both brakes, easing off the brakes as the cornering loads increase and avoiding sudden braking midcorner. Dragging the brakes with constant contact of pad on rim on long descents is bad practice that can result in carbon rim damage and/or tire failure. We will revisit this concept when we address cornering, a Level 2 skill (see page 165).

Countersteering

This skill is central to bike handling and is often overlooked. By applying a subtle forward pressure on the bar, you can initiate a turn, maintain a turning radius, change your chosen line, or ride a straight line while your bike is leaning to one side. Although it sounds complicated, countersteering is very natural movement that can open up a new world of control and confidence on a bike. If this skill is lacking, you cannot climb, corner, descend, or ride in the wind with optimal effect. Many riders already use this tool without actually being aware of it. Some may understand it, but most do not consciously apply it to their riding. Let's begin to apply it and use it to become a better rider.

PRACTICING COUNTERSTEERING

Find a flat section of road that is quiet and safe, and ride with your fingertips resting on the handlebars. Gently push forward on the right side of the handlebar. You will notice the wheel turns to the left, but the bike leans to the right and begins to "magically" turn right. This is countersteering.

Standing

Watch any triathlon race, or simply observe your training partners, and it will become very clear that many athletes are highly uncomfortable and inefficient at standing out of the saddle. This could be due to aggressive geometry or the setup of the time trial bike (or both), but more often it's user error. As we discussed earlier in the chapter, to stand effectively, you need to lean the bike toward the leg that is engaged in the downstroke of the pedal cycle, from 1 to 5 o'clock and countersteer to maintain a straight line. Standing out of the saddle requires coordination of pedaling cadence and the side-to-side motion of the bike. It is an evolution of the skill, but not a difficult one to learn.

Our sport is devoid of finish line sprints or sudden explosive efforts. Such exploits would come back to haunt a triathlete later in the event, as the energy cost would be greater than required to maintain needed momentum. Most triathlon courses require only brief efforts out of the saddle to gain, maintain, or regain momentum and to relieve postural stress. On occasion a course might include a very steep section of terrain, causing you to need to stand for more than 30 seconds. Manage the effort to keep it muscular and minimize the physiological cost. Standing up out of the saddle allows us to add our body weight to pedaling in an efficient and sustainable way. By transferring load between cardiovascular and muscular efforts, we create the potential to reduce stress and increase speed.

Standing becomes a powerful tool to maximize your speed potential while limiting cost; however, without skill development, each standing effort can be an energy drain or a momentum killer.

The pedal stroke changes when you get out of the saddle. The heel of the retreating leg leads the hip up and over the top of the pedal stroke, making for a bigger range of efficiency from 7 to 2 o'clock on the clock face. In other words, the more passive retreating leg becomes a very active and focused part of the pedal stroke. This action allows you to rise out of the saddle and propel your hip up over the pedal stroke.

PRACTICING STANDING

- Roll along at a relaxed pace, and gently lean the bike over. With the downstroking leg ready in the 1 o'clock position, transition to a bend at the waist, hip up, arms relaxed, light grip on the bars, looking ahead (note that the upper-body stance is very similar to the good posture you develop seated). Feel the counter-steering effort required to allow you to track straight without effort, then pause.
- Now complete the downstroke and smoothly lean the bike to the other side, pausing in this position, with the opposing leg in that 1 o'clock position. You are now set up with the other leg at the top of the stroke. Pause and repeat.
- Pausing between strokes allows you the time to check your form and ensure that you can gain feedback regarding your position and actions and how they affect the bike.
- Once you get a feel for the pause between strokes, move to fluid pedal strokes.

Good standing form cannot be trained on a conventional indoor trainer.

Now, we have established the role of the active retreating leg, but there's more. Leaning the bike in the direction of the downstroke will assist in getting the hip up over the pedal stroke. This action, combined with the lift as the leg retreats, allows you to straighten the leg and deploy body weight early (at 1 o'clock) in the front of the stroke, maximizing power. The final consideration

Cues for Efficient Pedaling While Standing

- Look ahead and plan where you want to go.
- Select a gear for resistance to pedal against.
- Rise up and forward.
- Bend at the waist.
- Draw the bike forward with the first strokes (from 7 to 2 o'clock).
- Use countersteering input.
- Lean the bike to assist the hip in coming up and over.
- Allow the bike to return to vertical without force.
- Straighten the leg early in the stroke.
- Keep hands supple, light on the handlebars.
- Maintain power from 4 to 8 o'clock.
- Control the heart rate.
- Keep standing efforts to 6 to 10 pedal strokes (each leg).
- Select the right gear to keep tension as you transition back.
- Return to the saddle and find a nice rhythm in seated riding.

is to subtly countersteer to allow the bike to hold a straight line despite leaning from side to side. (We will talk more about this topic later in the chapter.)

Remember that proper standing requires an efficient pedal stroke. Adding body weight to the action creates the need for a bigger "platform" to push against in order to maintain smooth, rhythmic riding (unless the grade of the hill shifts up dramatically). This means a heavier gear will be required, or you will be prone to sinking or blowing through the pedal stroke. By this, I mean that you are forced to overspin, or fail to have enough load, or tension on the chain, to allow proper mechanics to remain. Note that 80 percent of the momentum gained is in the first two pedal strokes. Once standing, 6 to 10 pedal strokes are typically all that is needed to maintain, gain, or create momentum. From there you must be careful to select the appropriate gear so that you can return to a seated position and regular pedaling without loss of momentum.

- There is no sudden load on the quads when you rise up.
- The contact patch of the tire, head, shoulders, and hips remains aligned at the center.
- The hands feel light.

- The tip of the saddle occasionally brushes the hamstring halfway between knee and buttock (as a result of leaning the bike).
- Heart rate does not climb much more than the few extra beats required to support your body weight.

And here are some indications that you aren't quite there yet:
- Sinking into the pedaling and wrestling the bike without a steady rhythm
- Failing to maintain a straight line
- Pressure of supporting the body weight being placed on the heels of the hands
- Losing momentum on returning to the saddle
- Heart rate, breathing, and/or perceived effort rocketing upward with each transition out of the saddle

---

CHECKING YOUR STANDING FORM

Simply ride the white line up a hill, with the sun behind you. If you are getting it right, the bike should track straight without steering. Watch your shadow on the road: There should be no up-and-down or side-to-side movement of the head and shoulders. Finally, your hands and handlebars should appear fluidly left and right of your torso.

LEVEL 2 | Interacting with the Terrain

Think of riding your bike as dancing with a swan rather than wrestling a pig. There are many pig wrestlers in triathlon! The inputs you need to get the bike to do what you want are both subtle and supple. The bike is your friend, and most of the time a well-designed bike will do what you want it to do if you don't get in the way of its natural tendencies. Knowing how to manage the wind, when to stand out of the saddle, and how to corner safely while maintaining speed will help you develop control and confidence on the bike.

Riding in the Wind

I approach this topic with fondness. In windy conditions, the ill-prepared perish and the well-prepared prevail. This is pure sport and an opportunity to show what you can do.

Admittedly, the sensation of being blown across the road or feeling as if your wheels might fly out from underneath you is unnerving. It causes tension in the upper body, disrupts pedaling rhythm, and in race situations often leads to catastrophic underfueling. It is very difficult to save energy, remain supple, and keep fueling if you are fighting to remain on the road. Your natural instinct is to counter the force of the wind by leaning into it, but ironically, this only makes it worse. Luckily, a few subtle changes will allow free-and-easy riding even in the most difficult conditions.

When riding in crosswinds, your initial focus should be on planning—anticipating when and where the wind will affect you. Look for gullies, gaps in trees, and exposed road features to anticipate gusts. Gauge wind direction and strength by observing the landscape around you—grass, trees, etc. Knowledge allows for better planning and management. What follows is a four-step process to help you relax, gain control, and maximize speed potential in the wind.

1. **Give yourself room.** If the wind is going to strike you from the left, then move more to the left of your lane (ensuring safety, of course).
2. **Gear up to gain greater control over your bike.** A slightly heavier gear will provide a more solid connection on the pedals. Once you settle in, you may be able to revert to a more normal gear, but use this heavier gear to gain control and comfort.
3. **Lean your bike away from the wind** (to the right if the wind is coming from the left). This requires a small countersteering effort on the right handlebar to maintain a straight line. This action is counterintuitive to most athletes, but you should point your wheels toward the wind and lean slightly away from it.
4. **Slide your butt slightly toward the wind and the center line of your bike** (to the left in this example) to maintain your center of balance. Maintain a supple upper body to allow the bike its natural self-correcting tendencies.

If you follow these steps, the wind will not get the best of you. To blow you across the road, it must overcome your steering slightly into the wind (the countersteering effect of riding straight while leaning to the right), and to blow the wheels from under you, it must lift your weight and move the wheels past the center line. It simply is not going to happen.

The final tip on riding in high winds is to fuel and hydrate on a regular timeline in order to set up a positive run. With the countersteering tool in effect, it is important that you eat and drink using the hand that is closest to the wind (the left hand in this example). This is one of the many reasons why learning to eat and drink with both hands is valuable.

Headwinds

In much the same way that you may struggle to make progress when climbing, spinning away with an uncomfortably high heart rate, it can be very challenging to ride into the wind. Learn to vary the cadence and load on the body to ride well. Having the postural fitness to maintain your best aero position for extended periods is essential.

Tailwinds

Having trained the ability to generate power with supple high-cadence pedaling, even after periods of higher muscular load, is key—and is especially important if a tailwind is accompanied by a gradual descent. Having appropriate gearing on your bike so that you are not spinning at an uncomfortably high rate certainly helps.

Riding Rolling Terrain

Any piece of terrain with positive and negative gradient that can be negotiated by gaining, maintaining, and regaining momentum without settling into a sustained climbing rhythm qualifies as a roller. There will be a slight increase in effort at the base and top of each roller, where there is the most to be gained, carrying momentum into the roller and accelerating over the top to carry those extra few miles per hour down the next section. Using muscle tension, roll a gear into the gradient carrying as much speed as practical before planning your downshifts to manage your effort through the body of the roller. This technique prepares your legs for the coming load. It helps you avoid the most frequent mistakes triathletes make on rollers—coasting into the gradient and from there suddenly loading up the legs or gearing down too far and going nowhere. If you do find yourself spinning, it can be solved by gearing back up and fluidly standing to regain momentum.

The extent of the rollers will determine the best approach. On soft or long crests, pick up speed through the gears and rebuild to race cadence. On hard or short crests, measured use of standing pedaling is particularly effective. Remember, the work is not done until you have built speed on the downslope. This approach gives you a colossal advantage over those who coast in and back off at their "mental summit."

PREPARING THE LEGS FOR LOAD

If you know that there will be a sudden increase in muscular load at the end of a period of high-cadence pedaling (e.g., a long descent followed by a steep rise), prepare the legs by introducing some higher-tension pedaling so as not to shock the body with a sudden change of load.

Cornering

Cornering skill and speed are best built by banking positive and controlled experiences, not by riding on the edge of your ability and inducing fear. My objective is to help you corner safely and with confidence, allowing plenty of margin for little mistakes. Let's get a better understanding of how cornering plays out.

Cornering speed on a bike is limited by traction and the speed at which you are able to come out of the corner. Traction is influenced by tire selection and pressure, road surface, camber, the lean angle of the bike, and braking force. Most good race tires have a similar amount of grip, but problems arise if the tire is overinflated for your body weight or the road conditions. The manufacturer's inflation recommendations are a good place to start, but note that the maximum recommended pressure will reduce the tire's grip and even add to rolling resistance in many circumstances. Road surface—both the texture and whatever is on it, such as dust or water—determines the amount of available traction. Furthermore, the camber of the road determines the relative lean angle of the bike—the greater the camber, the smaller the relative lean angle will be to maintain traction. In the traction equation, we obviously can't exceed 100 percent of available traction. So if you use 50 percent of available traction for braking, then demand 60 percent of the traction for turning, problems will arise! This is why you should have much or all of your braking completed before you initiate the turn of the corner and have other options than braking midcorner.

So how do we get it *right*? Once again, be aware and have a plan. When driving on the highway, you watch for the exit signs so as to avoid cutting across four lanes at the last moment, and it's the same on the bike. Shift your attention forward and gather information continually. For example, while descending, take the opportunity to look several corners ahead so that you can notice a narrow, decreasing-radius corner three turns ahead. Store this information and formulate a plan. This means you will have less information to process and more time to do it when approaching that corner.

Many triathletes use one of the two cornering options every time, whether it's a conscious decision or habit. A better understanding of how and when to execute all three, and especially the late-apex, will transform your riding, making you more confident and increasing your enjoyment of descents. See Figure 7.4 to learn more about the three lines you can take on a corner.

Braking & Cornering

With the current generation of road brakes, it's hard to exceed the available traction when riding in a straight line on a dry road. When cornering, it's a much more precarious situation. If the bike is a few degrees off or the friction at the contact patch is compromised even a little, the available traction can easily and inadvertently be exceeded. There is more braking force available at the front wheel due to weight distribution; however, as a general rule, you should apply the brakes evenly, with progressive force. Less-confident riders should try to finish braking before cornering—it's the safest protocol, but it's a little slower. As cornering confidence builds, you can maintain more speed by easing off the brakes as cornering load increases. Be aware that proper braking protocol on long descents requires that you apply the brakes and release them to moderate speed. Dragging the brakes constantly on the rim can lead to tire or rim failure. Here are some pointers for safely navigating corners.

Don't strangle the bike. A controlled but relaxed grip on the bars leads to smooth, quick reactions and allows the bike to self-correct. Maintain your riding posture while cornering—fingers relaxed, wrists straight, elbows flexed, and neck and shoulders relaxed. Know when to leave the bike alone—don't fight it.

Keep head and eyes turned in the direction you want to go. The body naturally follows in the direction you are looking. To work on this, you can overcompensate at first; turning your head farther in the desired direction is a good way to condition yourself to avoid that sideways glance at the tree or lamppost on the outside of the curve.

FIGURE 7.4 ⋮ CORNERING

1. INSIDE

This is the shortest distance around the corner and is most often used on broad, constant, or opening-radius curves that allow maximum speed.

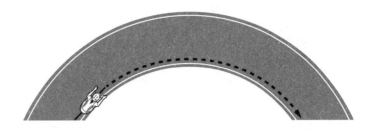

2. CLASSIC OUTSIDE-INSIDE-OUTSIDE

From the outside edge of the available lane, the arc cuts close to the inside radius in the middle of the corner and exits the turn close to the outside of the available lane. It's called "classic" because it is the line most commonly used.

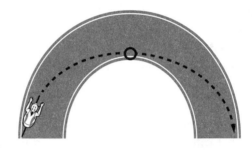

3. LATE-APEX

For decreasing-radius corners or those where the exit is obscured, the line begins wide and runs deeper into the corner before we release the brakes and initiate the turn past the center of the corner.

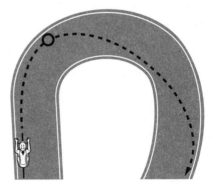

For decreasing-radius turns, initiating the turn and turning in happens over a shorter distance with slightly greater load on the front tire, so it is best practice to be off the brakes when turning in.

Keep weight on the outside pedal. This adds vertical force, pushing the bike down into the road. Body position should be low and centered over the bike.

Initiate the turn. A countersteering input on the inside handlebar is all it takes to initiate the turn. In a cambered corner, the initial input may be all that is required; then you can relax and allow the bike to follow the curve. In a flat, off-camber or decreasing-radius curve, a subtle or gently increasing input may be required.

Position your knee. In fast corners with good traction, the knee can be kept in and the bike bent down toward it. In some corners, initially pointing the inside knee and shoulder toward the inside of the turn draws the bike around. Keeping the bike more upright, pointing the knee, and leaning the body inward sets up less shear angle and is useful in wet or low-traction situations.

If your initial cornering plan was solid, these pointers are all that is required to maintain your chosen line. By entering a corner with a margin of error built into your plan, you will avoid emergencies, but sometimes the plan needs to change because of other riders, road debris, or obstacles at your chosen exit. First, do a quick check that your posture is good—most importantly, that your head and eyes are pointed where you want to end up. Once again, countersteering is your primary means of changing the path your bike is following—with a little more countersteering input, the bike will follow a tighter line. To steer around the outside of an obstacle, stand the bike up a little and then reapply countersteering. Braking midcorner should be your last resort.

Checkpoints for Better Cornering

The answers to these questions should help you choose the right line:

- Where is the exit?
- Where is the apex?
- Where are you going to initiate the turn?
- Where are you going to finish braking?
- Where will you need to start braking?

Practice applying different lines and cornering techniques on safe, familiar roads or vacant parking lots to build experience and recognize the options. This can be as simple as rolling up to a suburban intersection, planning the corner, turning the head and eyes, relaxing over the center of the bike, weighting the outside pedal, countersteering, shifting gear, rising up out of the saddle, smoothly accelerating, and transitioning back to seated pedaling. Speed will build naturally without you having to chase it, force it, or compromise your safety—you will execute your plan more easily and go faster.

Cornering, like most of the other bike-handling skills discussed in this chapter, requires neuromuscular conditioning, which takes time and attention. Focus on these skills early in the season to build good habits and techniques that can be developed, honed, and carried forward into racing to maximize performance.

A FINAL WORD ON RIDING AWARENESS

For the vast majority of triathletes, Level 3 riding is not relevant. If you have not mastered your interaction with the bike and the application of your skills to the terrain, you probably do not yet have the tools to impose yourself on others on the course. Thinking about your competitors will only be a distraction and therefore counterproductive to achieving your best race outcome. A smart racer will be influenced by the competition—that is, change the race plan—only if such a reaction provides a clear benefit.

The majority of your time on most courses will be spent meting out your trained potential in your most aerodynamic position. But note that even if only 5 percent of the course requires that your time be spent deploying other tactics (or "tools," as we like to call them), real and significant advantage can be gained. Training the most basic interactions with your bike and building the resilience and confidence to properly apply them will allow you to maximize the bike and bring your best form to the run.

Consciously practice your skills every time you ride. The beginning of any ride should always be used to check your riding tools and establish good habits—attention to form at the end of the ride is critical to performance and allows us to bank those positive sensations and build on them. An added bonus of developing your riding skills and tools is the simple pleasure of having ridden well regardless of the numbers.

TRAINING THE BIKE IN TRIATHLON

I am often asked which of the three sports is most important to work on; in answer, I remind athletes that triathlon should always be viewed as one sport: swim-bike-run. Nonetheless, I think it is safe to say that riding conditioning and training should be at the center of preparation for most triathletes. Cycling is the discipline that takes the most time to complete, and one that can yield great performance results with consistent application. Finally, the effectiveness of your riding ability has implications that carry over to your running potential off the bike. For all these reasons, dedicated athletes cannot overlook the need to develop strong and resilient cycling.

As I have mentioned before, all of your riding should carry a purpose within the fabric of your training day and training week. This doesn't mean that it should all be at the same level of intensity or in pursuit of the same goal. In fact, the range of intensity associated with a solid cycling training plan is perhaps wider than that of any other discipline. As in most endurance sports, real progression and performance development require significant time on the bike, and I like to remind athletes that it is important to set up your riding training to maximize riding performance gains in a single season and facilitate riding evolution over multiple seasons. Including specific focus in the sessions within each phase will allow progression and an opportunity for continued success—but it takes time.

What are we aiming to train and improve when we repeat weeks and weeks of consistent training?

Cardiovascular fitness. Because cycling is a lower-impact sport, it allows extended duration of training load without massive consequence.

Muscular resilience. This is key to maintaining speed late in the race, and it also allows good running off the bike.

Technical efficiency. Some of the training and intervals are designed to improve your brain's ability to talk to the muscles, also known as motor programming. Improved muscle sequencing reduces the physiological cost under a given workload, allowing for longer efforts.

Sustainable power. This process begins with improving power potential into high power, then transforming that power into greater sustainable power over extended durations. In other words, you don't just want to lower cost, you want to transform your energy savings into going fast for longer periods.

Let's now focus on the training: how much riding, how often, what types of sessions, and how to structure a season of progression for performance development and race readiness.

Setting Up Your Year

As with discussions of swimming and running, I have to begin with the obvious caveat that one approach does not fit every situation and athlete. In any given season, I have athletes with progressions and phases of training that are not synchronized with the outline that follows, but this approach fits the majority of Northern Hemisphere athletes. Within the scope of this progression, there is plenty of room to shift the focus to work on a rider's specific weaknesses or needs, but the overall outline will culminate in an extended phase of training for the specific demands of your event.

Post-season Bike Training

Reduced training stress
Emphasis on technique

This is the time to enjoy plenty of lower-intensity and less structured riding—it can still help you evolve.

This phase delivers the lowest training stress from an emotional and physiological standpoint, but it holds critical value in the overall season progression. Use this time to focus on the technical aspects of cycling with the goal of developing foundational cardiovascular endurance and improving the effectiveness of your pedal stroke. In my coaching, I often refer to cycling stress, or load, being placed "upstairs or downstairs" to help the athlete nail down the mission of the session or intervals. "Upstairs" refers to cardiovascular stress, "downstairs" to a more muscular load. Of course there is always a balance of stressors in normal riding, but we weight our focus according to the training phase or session goals. In the post-season, load is focused upstairs, with an emphasis on foundational fitness, neurological programming, and lighter sessions. Any focus downstairs is for the purposes of muscular recruitment and pedaling improvements. The post-season will seldom include high stress upstairs and downstairs at the same time. We tend to think about stressing each in isolation in order to keep overall training load low. The post-season is a great opportunity to change up the type of cycling you do. Hopping on the road bike, or even a 'cross or mountain bike, provides emotional relief from the highly structured race season, and it's also a great way to work on handling. With plenty of time before the key races, the post-season is the best time to focus on bike handling and skills.

HIGH-CADENCE INTERVALS

To improve the dialogue between your brain and the riding muscles, include intervals at low power and high cadence. The stress here is upstairs. Focus on maintaining fluid pedal strokes and relaxed upper body.

Warm-up	**15–30 min.** low intensity Z2
Pre–Main Set	**6 to 10 × 2 min.,** no breaks
	Build cadence every 30 sec. (75, 85, 95, 105 rpm)
Main Set	**4 × 3 min., 4 × 2 min., 4 × 1 min., 4 × 30 sec., 4 × 1 min., 4 × 2 min., 4 × 3 min.**
	All highest rpm you can hold at Z1/2 to Z2 power
	Between each interval ride 1 min. smooth Z2 choice rpm with great form.
	Then ride home Z2 to Z2/3 with as good form and pedal stroke as you can.

MUSCLE TENSION INTERVALS

Shift the load downstairs with low- to medium-power muscle-tension work. You should be able to maintain relaxed breathing and lower heart rates, as this session is pure muscle recruitment and form. If you complete intervals on a hill, the grade should be shallow (4 to 6 percent) and relatively consistent. Focus on the retreating leg and the 5 to 11 o'clock part of the stroke to develop balanced recruitment and great tension on the chain.

Warm-up	15–30 min. low intensity Z2
Pre–Main Set	**5, 4, 3, 2, 1 min.**
	All Z2/3 building rpm from as slow as you can hold with smooth pedal stroke up to fast rpm
	Recover with 30 sec. Z1 between each interval.
Main Set	**6 × 5 min., 5 × 4 min., 4 × 3 min., 2 × 2 min., 1 × 1 min.**
	All Z2/3 to Z3 with as slow rpm as you can hold seated with fluid and even pedal stroke.
	Recover with 1 min. Z1/2 fast pedaling with no bounce between intervals.
	Then ride home Z2 to Z2/3 with as good form and pedal stroke as you can.

The rest of the riding in each week will be more endurance-focused but may well include elements of these sessions or a bigger skills component. It is easy to include some skills-based and technique-based riding within any given endurance ride, with high cadence/low power or bigger-gear muscle-tension work possibly becoming the focus of an extended ride. The additional rides of the week are a great opportunity to work on many of the skills and focus points we discussed in regard to becoming a better rider earlier in the chapter. Once a week you could have the freedom to ride your mountain bike or 'cross bike, but safety and smart riding rules.

Pre-season Bike Training

Post-season riding allows us to absorb the heavier training that begins in this phase of the year. Endurance, strength, and (sometimes) high power make up the backbone of the weekly sessions.

For most developing athletes, the pre-season phase begins with the start of the year, marking a shift to a much greater training load. This is the phase in which the bulk of cardiovascular and muscular endurance is established. The goal of this phase is simple: Build strength, endurance, and muscular resilience in pursuit of power potential. In this phase, you experience a real development of fitness and improved strength. A very experienced athlete who has trained for years and established great foundational fitness could focus on power development as a route to a performance jump later in the season. Consequently, there would be less focus on general conditioning. For both developing and experienced athletes, there is heavy emphasis on muscular recruitment and strength in this phase, with low-cadence, medium-effort intervals included once or twice in weekly training.

MUSCLE-TENSION WORK

We progress the recruitment work of the post-season and increase the load both upstairs and downstairs, with strength-based muscle tension or hill repetitions. Most athletes are in the high-strength phase of functional strength training at this time, and the hill work, or low cadence, is a perfect companion. The overall load is still focused on riding muscles, and breathing/heart rate should still be load. At this tension/power, we can also include some technical standing practice in the intervals.

Warm-up	**30–60 min.** low intensity Z2
Pre–Main Set	**2–3 rounds of progressive 1-min. intervals:**
	1 min. Z2/3, 1 min. Z3, 1 min. Z3/4, 1 min. Z4, 1 min. Z4/5. All fast cadence (for most riders 95–110 rpm)
	30 sec. Z1 recovery after each interval
	Follow the set with 2 min. easy spin.
	We just touch some higher-end work to ensure that the neuromuscular system is awake. This prepares us for the work ahead.
Main Set	**6 × 8–10 min.** Z3 to Z3+ at low cadence
	Focus on steady and consistent tension on the chain with 8–10 pedal strokes standing with perfect transitions when terrain tips up, or every third minute.
	Spin down easy between each interval.
	Then ride home Z2 to Z2/3 with good form and a smooth pedal stroke.

TENSION-VARIANCE ENDURANCE WORK

A second endurance-based strength workout includes cadence variance at a similar power. The transition between cadences while climbing allows shifting pedal strokes, muscular recruitment, and a solid platform for beginning to develop increased power in the pedal stroke.

Warm-up	**30–60 min.** low intensity Z2
Pre–Main Set	**6 to 8 × 3 min.,** progress effort in sets of two
	Ride the last two strong and consistent with great rhythm and good form.
	Recover 1–2 min. between each interval. No zones, just an extended warm-up with focus on form through progressive intensity.
Main Set	**2 to 5 × 8–20 min.** Z3/Z3+
	Ride 2 min. seated at slow cadence, then 2 min. spinning faster rpm in lighter gear, continuous throughout each climb.
	Focus on steady, consistent tension on the chain in the seated climbing sections, then hold that form when cadence rises and you are in a lighter gear. The slow cadence should be in a bigger gear than you would naturally select, the faster cadence in a smaller gear than is natural.
	Finish with one more interval of the same duration, all with your most natural and effective cadence and pedaling.
	This should result in great form, comfort, and your highest power/speed on the final interval.
	Then ride home Z2 to Z2/3 with as good form and pedal stroke as you can.

RECOVERY

As in the post-season, most of the rest of your weekly rides are form-based endurance rides. With this increase in overall training stress in this part of the season, you will likely add in some lower-stress prep rides or recovery rides. It is absolutely critical that you keep the lower-stress endurance riding very easy, almost all Z2 or under. For many, this means the vast bulk of total riding in each training block is Z2 or under.

Warm-up	15–30 min. light spinning in very easy gear
Pre–Main Set	3 × 10 min. Z1/2 light gear and faster spinning
	Minutes 3, 6, 9 are Z2/3, Z3, Z3/4, respectively, to open the pipes and force blood flow.
	Then done.

PREP-RIDE

Warm-up	15–30 min. light spinning in very easy gear
Pre–Main Set	4 to 6 × 2 min., ride as:
	30 sec. Z2 at 80 rpm, 30 sec. Z2/3 at 90 rpm, 1 min. Z3 at 90+ rpm
Main Set	2 to 4 × 6 min., build by 2 min. to the last 2 min. at Z2/3 to Z3
	Focus on rhythm riding and good form.
	Then ride home, easy spinning with lighter gear.

Sustained Power Bike Training

Remember that these are the key sessions, and lower-intensity endurance and skills-based sessions will support these main sessions within a week.

This is often the shortest phase of training over the course of the season. It is really an opportunity to "sharpen" the fitness gained in the early phases of the season. The key weekly sessions include a greater focus on very-high-intensity training, which by extension results in a drop in weekly riding hours. That said, plenty of athletes have been waiting out a cold winter, and when they are finally able to get outside, they will likely want to ride more. Early-season races often accompany this phase of the year, serving as great opportunities to continue to build resilience and begin to get race-fit.

BUILDING SUSTAINED POWER

I like to set athletes up for success in higher-intensity sessions, especially when I consider the session as part of the fabric of the entire training week. To do this, I often design interval-based sessions to be progressive building efforts. In addition to the success factor, it facilitates pacing and building focus, which are key for race performance for most athletes. Note that this session is a key piece of building sustainable power, yet too many athletes fail to hit this type of intensity.

If you wish to improve your maximal steady state (FTP) then don't spend too much training time sitting right around that power, instead, complete intervals above this output, as follows.

Warm-up	**15–45 min.** smooth build
Pre–Main Set	**2 to 3 × 9 min.** Z2 Ride minutes 3, 6, 9 as Z3, Z3/4, Z4, respectively.
Main Set	**8 × 6 min.** 1–4: Progress from 1 to 4 to *very strong* (Z5). *Check power on 4.* 5–8: Maintain the power achieved on fourth set of building efforts. 5 min. easy riding between each interval *If you begin to fail in the later intervals, then maintain power and trim interval length by 1 min. Maintain the same rest interval.*

SUSTAINED POWER

I believe in *variance* as a great component of adaptation and of forcing stimulus to evolve. I also like athletes to *think* their way through sessions and be forced to shift both effort (power) and cadence (rate of pedal stroke) within a session. This is a great stimulator of improving maximal sustainable power by dancing under, at, and just above the power/effort of your most efficient pedal stroke.

Warm-up	**15–45 min.** smooth and easy spinning
Pre–Main Set	**6 × 3 min.** continuous, ride as 30 sec. Z1, 30 sec. Z2, 1 min. Z3, 30 sec. Z3/4, 30 sec. Z4 Then 5–10 min. easy spin.

Main Set	5 to 7 continuous rounds:
	6 min. Z3 to Z3/4 choice/most efficient pedal stroke
	4 min. Z4 most efficient pedal stroke plus 5 rpm
	2 min. Z4/5 most efficient pedal stroke plus 5 to 7 rpm
	1 min. complete recovery Z1
	3 min. easy spinning Z1/2

Race-Specific Bike Training

If you were preparing for a later-season Ironman race such as Hawaii or Arizona, you might transition into race specificity in May, but the emotional or physical shift to Ironman mode would wait. Your initial race-specific focus would likely be around your midseason shorter races (typically Ironman 70.3 distance). Following a midseason break, you would rebuild and transition to a full A-goal Ironman focus 9 to 14 weeks prior to the race day.

The longest phase of the season is often a split phase for year-round triathletes. Toward the end of April, it's likely that you have progressed through a more relaxed post-season, built pre-season conditioning, and even hit a few weeks of higher-intensity and lower-volume power and speed. With a few early-season races under your belt, you arrive at this phase with good overall fitness and power potential but not specifically trained for the key events of the season—fit and strong yet not race-ready. The race-specific phase often means a fork in the road, depending on the length of your key events. Shorter-distance athletes experience sustained intensity with the training session, but longer-distance athletes turn their focus to building great resilience and readiness to hold medium-intensity efforts for extended periods.

In your riding, you want to focus not just on the demands of the distance you are training for but also on the specifics of the course and conditions you expect to face. Experienced athletes and pros will also prepare for different potential race dynamics. "Race specificity" is the phrase to remember here, as all key sessions serve as dress rehearsals for race day. The more practice we put in, close to race specificity, the more habitual the whole experience becomes—and you will arrive at the starting line prepared.

The simple goal of this part of the season is to train for the demands and distance of your event. In addition, you should consider the actual course you are preparing for: the likely weather conditions and the terrain. These factors can help you tailor your preparation in this part of the season. As for swimming and running, we aim to build the key cycling sessions as dress rehearsals for the big day. There is a physical familiarization in this training to prepare but also an emotional familiarization with what you expect to experience on race day. If you build specific conditioning, can simulate the race experience, and gain confidence in the process, then race day will be more habitual for you. It always amazes me that athletes simply ride their bikes a long way on the weekend instead becoming trained and familiar with the sensations that accompany riding under, at, and just above race intensity. Let's look at examples of typical key bike sessions for the three main distances in the sport: Olympic, Ironman 70.3, and Ironman.

OLYMPIC RACE-SPECIFIC SESSIONS

There are dozens of short-course-specific sessions that we might employ, with many variations for different levels of athletes. Let's assume this session is for nondrafting athletes, who are less influenced by other athletes in the race. This session is focused on maintaining high sustainable effort in a relaxed fashion while under duress.

Warm-up	20–40 min. easy riding
Pre–Main Set	4 × 2 min., progress 1 to 4 to Z3/4 4 × 1 min., progress 1 to 4 to Z4 4 × 30 sec., progress 1 to 4 to Z4/5 All with 30 sec. easy between intervals
Main Set	**2 to 4 rounds:** **4 to 8 × 1 min.** Z4/5 fast rpm, with 30 sec. easy between intervals **8 to 12 min.** maximal steady state Z4+ In the last 2–4 min. add 5–7 rpm and maintain power/effort/speed. All with great riding with relaxed form. Ride 7–10 min. easy between rounds.

If this workout is completed correctly, with very-high-intensity shorter intervals, you should feel under duress in the early part of each interval but settle to a very strong and sustainable effort as the steady state continues.

IRONMAN 70.3 RACE-SPECIFIC SESSIONS

As for the Ironman-specific sessions below, I want athletes to spend a great deal of time getting familiar just under, at, and above race-specific intensity. This session builds effort and intensity to train you to have a greater capacity for duress on the back end of the session, which is where we hope your best riding will occur during the race. It takes massive focus on pacing to execute these progressive intervals. If you blow up, it is a good reminder to listen to your body and pace your effort based on what you have in the tank on a given day.

When you exit the swim on race day, the transition involves several minutes of running and changing. In training, I like my athletes to hop on the bike after a short run to get familiar with this sensation so they can adapt faster.

	Run 10 min. smooth
	Build effort with good leg speed.
Warm-up	**15–45 min.** easy spinning
Pre–Main Set	**4 × 3 min.**, progress each as Z2, Z3, Z3/4 with faster rpm
Main Set	**1 × 30 min.**, ride as 15 min. under 70.3 pace, 15 min. at race pace
	2 × 25 min., ride as 5 min. under 70.3 pace, 15 min. at race pace, 5 min. above pace
	3 × 20 min., ride as 15 min. at 70.3 pace, 5 min. above race pace
	All with 5–7 min. easy spinning between each interval.

IRONMAN-SPECIFIC SESSIONS

There is a general obsession with distance in Ironman training. While there is great value in some extended-duration rides that are closer to or above the 112-mile race distance, the Ironman-specific rides fall short of that distance, lasting 4 to 4.5 hours (75 to 90 miles for the elite crowd). In this example, we focus on extended sustained efforts just under, at, and above Ironman race intensity. In addition, we again simulate the race-day experience and goals when first getting onto the bike and the preparation to run following the bike.

When you exit the swim on race day, there are several minutes of running and changing. I like my athletes to hop on the bike after a short run to get familiar with this sensation so they can adapt faster.

	Run 10 min. around Ironman race effort with good leg speed
Warm-up	30 min. easy at faster-than-usual rpm
	Hold cadence a little higher in the initial stages of the bike race, then fall into natural rhythm.
Main Set	6 × 40 min. as 5 min. under race pace, 25 min. at race pace, 10 min. at or above race pace with slightly higher cadence
	Recover with 10 min. easy spinning between 40-min. intervals.
	Manage the effort throughout the interval to do your best riding at the end of the interval, which prepares you to finish strong on race day. The cadence play is neurological training to enable you to maintain cadence in the final quarter of the ride. Cadence typically falls in that quarter, to the detriment of wheel speed and setting up for a good run.
Additional Set	10–30 min. Ride at or above Ironman race-pace intensity with the goal of holding cadence just above your norm.
	This is a big final stimulus to emotionally prepare you for the upcoming run section. This takes practice and rehearsal.

TRAINING YOUR TRANSITIONS

Triathlon riding begins at the end of the swim, and your run begins before the end of the ride. Sustainable effort and pacing in the controlled anarchy of racing is an art that requires the wisdom of experience, but also training.

Racing entails sensations that many athletes never experience in training. On race day, you have the additional factors of spectators, other competitors, nutrition, course markers, and heightened anticipation. In addition, you ride your bike after a genuine race-effort swim and transition and also have to maximize your run performance following a race-effort bike. These new sensations can take up a great amount of focus and emotional energy unless you train yourself to become so familiar with them that coping with them becomes an ingrained habit by race day.

There are very real mechanical applications to help you settle and find your "riding legs" when getting on your bike as well as applications that can help prepare you physically while still on the bike to run well. Below is a list of skills and habits to develop in the race-specific phase of training to ensure that you are not just fit but race-ready.

We don't always need to ride following a tough swim, as we can't always get to a pool on demand, and a short run before the ride can elevate heart rate and simulate the cost of a transition run. The result of short pre-ride runs is familiarization with the heavy legs you will feel when mounting the bike on race day.

Early riding. When you first get on the bike on race day, there *will* be a period when the brain is not quite "talking" to the legs. We want to hasten the discussion and drive blood to the working tissues so you can find your riding groove. In the early stages of a ride, I like to see athletes go one gear lighter (not too light, just a touch lighter) with a slightly faster cadence. As the legs begin to feel like riding legs, you begin to find rhythm and fall into natural form and cadence flow.

Midcourse riding. While the aerodynamic time trial position is fast, it is counterproductive for a tall, proud running form. Throughout a training or race ride, I like to see riders shift the load on their bodies and stretch the lower back and hips. Gearing up and transitioning out of the saddle, then stretching the lower back (by keeping the hips straight but turning your shoulders from side to side) and pushing the hips forward may feel like a time loss, but it is an investment in your readiness to run. You've got to give a little to run well off the bike!

End of the ride. It is important that you prepare physically and emotionally for the second transition and run portions of the race. Revert to one lighter gear over any rollers, push one lighter gear on any downhill phases that require big effort, and generally reengage the neurological programming, effectively returning to the style of riding used for the first part of the bike leg. In addition to this faster cadence, you might stretch the back and hips a few times throughout the last miles to ensure that you can transition to good running posture as quickly as possible. This is where you will experience a massive performance bonus if you are set up in a great sustainable bike fit and you have developed strong postural fitness. The final piece of the puzzle is emotional focus. You should rehearse your transition protocol in your head—the layout, order of events, and running out of the transition zone with good form—supple, relaxed—and fast feet. Don't hop off the bike in a panic; I want you to transition off the bike with purpose. It sounds rudimentary, but I promise that most athletes don't think about it, and fewer actually train for it. This isn't about faster transitions. It is about making transitions seamless and preserving your priceless physical and emotional resources.

SETTING UP A WORKOUT

Riding requires specificity in any given session in order to yield optimal gains. A typical session, on the road or on the trainer, would progress as:

Warm-up. Always prepare the body for the work ahead. A period of low-intensity, light spinning gets the brain "talking" to the muscles and begins to raise your body temperature and increase blood flow to the muscles. It is a great time to focus on riding skills, cadence play, or handling skills, so warm-up time isn't without purpose. Some athletes require more warm-up than others to be ready for high-quality work. It's important to develop an understanding of what works best for you.

If you always feel flat in initial intervals of a session and improve as you go on, you may not be getting an adequate warm-up.

Pre–main set. When riding outside, there is seldom a pause between the warm-up and the pre–main set, but there will likely be a shift in focus, depending on the type of ride you are doing. For an endurance ride, you may shift to some higher-cadence work. For a little neurological training, complete some light building efforts from easy to a stronger workload. Either way, the focus of this part of the workout is often technical or skills-based. You should finish the pre–main set primed for the main set and riding with great form.

Main set. You are now ready for focused intervals. This set can range from extended hours at Ironman effort to easy spinning with high cadence for recovery. Either way, the main set will make up at least 70 percent of your overall riding time.

Following the main set, there is seldom more specific work. The occasional *additional set* might be appropriate and will be power-based technique or pure endurance riding. Either way, there is little need for a massive warm-down and certainly no time for mindless riding. Any riding following a main set should be performed with focus on good form and a possible shift in mind-set to running off the bike.

8

Running in Triathlon

Because running is the third sport completed on race day, it is where most issues rear their ugly heads. Nearly all nutritional disasters, cramping, blow-ups, and exhaustion occur during the running portion of the race. This cruel reality can lead to some confusion, especially following a poor race result. I cannot count the number of times I have been told by frustrated triathletes that they really need to "work on their running" after a poor running performance in a race. This may be true, but poor running preparation is often not the culprit in a poor run performance. Running performance is always influenced by what precedes it in the race—the swim and the bike. If there is ever a need to remember that the sport is swim-bike-run—not swimming, biking, and running—this is the time.

Considered within the context of the sport as a whole, running seems to receive the least critical thought or review in terms of training, form, or progression. Perhaps this is because running is the most intuitive and familiar of the disciplines. Nearly all triathletes have *some* running history, even if it was only keep-fit jogging. So when racing disasters repeatedly occur within the run segment, it is easy for triathletes to fall into a "more is better" approach.

Running is also the king of injury. It's the most corrosive of the three triathlon disciplines because it is fully weight-bearing and is therefore the predominant cause of muscular damage. For many athletes, training and racing are compromised by a cycle of injuries directly or indirectly caused by running. There is little doubt that many injuries are triggered by one or a combination of:

- Run training load that has progressed too aggressively
- Poor running mechanics, especially when fatigued
- Inadequate musculoskeletal integrity to sustain training load

As with any sport, training load is a combination of frequency, intensity (how hard), and duration (commonly known as volume). It is important to distinguish, or at least consider, your volume or duration both in terms of accumulated running over a period and the duration of single running sessions. In other words, *how you accumulate volume* has a significant effect on injury risk or occurrence.

The typical approach to run training has been influenced by the fear-based goal of trying to prevent the catastrophic events that plague so many athletes on race day. High mileage and a strong focus on the long run have become the staples of most triathlon training programs, particularly those focusing on longer-distance events. "Run, and run some more" is the mantra, yet the same problems persist, and fatigue-laden running is the norm. We have to ask the question: Are we going about run training the right way?

It's my belief that *too many bad footsteps* are taken in triathlon running. I am not suggesting that every triathlete strive for perfect running biomechanics. Many athletes direct their focus toward accumulating running miles and give little attention to ensuring that the miles they do complete are run with their best form and designed to yield positive results. This leaves countless enthusiasts to slog through training sessions with poor form, battling fatigue, increasing their risk of injury, achieving high levels of muscle damage and fatigue, and gaining a limited return from their training efforts.

When athletes equate miles with success, their training time typically lacks specificity, with little differentiation between specific sessions—or much else, for that matter. The lack of specificity that dominates many running programs is made worse by a lack of focus on looking after the body from a functional standpoint and setting it up to withstand the great load that running places on the musculoskeletal system. We have athletes who are weak and lack mobility in the joints and thus are unable to withstand a proper training load without injury. Despite these common issues, athletes tend to place little to no value on a complementary progressive functional strength and mobility training program. Any strength-based program is typically jettisoned as soon as the season heats up in order to accommodate more running in the weekly schedule.

DEBUNKING THE MYTHS OF TRIATHLON RUNNING

MYTH: **The long run is key.** When it comes to Ironman-distance racing, many triathletes worry over whether they will be "fit enough" on the run. The distance of the event creates fear, and most triathletes respond by running distances close to the race distance each week. Unfortunately, this approach places too much emphasis on the long run, which is the most corrosive of all sessions in terms of the muscular damage it causes. Furthermore, it often has the greatest negative impact on the following days of training. Consistency and improved muscle resilience are the best preparation for the run portion of the race. Frequency is more important—and less risky—than any single session. Some extended-duration sessions are helpful, but don't pin all your dreams and hopes on them.

MYTH: **Functional strength is not important.** The vast majority of triathletes have relatively limited neuromuscular awareness, strength, balance, and power-creating potential. Functional strength is *not* a replacement for running, nor does it guarantee injury-free training, but it will help establish the foundational strength required to maximize the specific run training you do. It is not a question of whether you can "get away" without strength and conditioning training—such training is key in your continual evolution as an athlete.

MYTH: **Running form or technique cannot be improved, so just run.** Too many coaches and athletes overlook form and technical improvements. While it's true that you do not need to run like an elite runner, there are simple areas of focus that can help improve form and economy, regardless of your level of performance. Any of these technical improvements may seem minor because they are mostly about the mind-set that will help you keep moving effectively, but they still call for focus and attention.

MYTH: **All runs must be hard or strong.** If you aren't breaking down the doors of the barn, how are you improving? One of the biggest mistakes I see triathletes make is performing nearly all of their runs at moderately hard to hard effort. Little time is spent at very low intensity, and, ironically, this prevents athletes from being able to hit a very high intensity. Effective run training will have a large divergence between high and low intensity. Embrace running easy, but learn to do so while maintaining an effective foot speed.

MYTH: **It is impossible to make great improvements in running.** As with swimming, too many athletes declare themselves to be poor runners and resign themselves to plodding through races. Improved running requires a true commitment (more than a few months) to evolving form, strength, and focus, but it can be achieved.

MYTH: **Lighter body weight is always better.** This is a highly disruptive and risky myth. If you can be as light as possible while still maintaining your power and hormonal health, then great, but that is not typically how it goes. Most athletes resort to restricting calories or employing other weight-loss strategies that result in increased risk of injury; a disruption of hormonal balance; and, following initial success, weakness and fatigue. If getting lighter is necessary, it should be a part of a complete approach to the sport, not a means to an end.

MYTH: **You must run on the forefoot.** I see many athletes running around on tiptoe. This stems from the idea that the best way to improve technique is to get onto the front of the foot. Unfortunately, when athletes land on their toes rather than their forefoot, it greatly heightens the load and stress on the Achilles tendon and calf muscles. Injury can result. Believe it or not, many highly successful runners happen to land on the midfoot to back of the foot (the heel) and still transfer to the ball of the foot quickly, without increased load. Don't try to control the landing of your foot; it will evolve as your run training, form, and strength progress. In other words, foot strike is typically *not a focus* when it comes to improving form.

MYTH: **Running form is highly technical and requires video analysis.** Although the technical aspects of running are important, don't immediately conclude that you have to spend lots of money and time on a detailed video analysis, especially if the resulting recommendations will be focused on fine motor movements. Instead, get the key principles correct, using simple cues and plenty of training. Don't be blinded by the details of perfect running form. If you try to run like Usain Bolt, you will surely fail. There are too many details to be implemented, which overcomplicates technique relative to what you are trying to achieve. Furthermore, pure running form has close to zero application when it comes to running well off the bike.

MYTH: **Injuries are just a part of running.** Injury risk should be greater for those truly pushing the boundaries of the sport—the pros! As an amateur, you don't have to be injured. While running is inherently risky, a careful, long-term approach will radically reduce the severity and frequency of overuse injuries.

MYTH: **Most triathlon run performance issues can be attributed to a lack of run training.** This one's my favorite. If you struggle with running off the bike, don't automatically double your run training. Remember that triathlon is swim-bike-run. Your run performance is related to your run training but also to your swim and bike training, your race execution (or pacing), your fueling approach, the fatigue you bring into the race, and your emotional energy expended up to that point of the race. Consider each factor before adapting your approach.

BONUS MYTH: **Running must always be at the center of triathlon weekly training for progression.** Running is the one discipline that tends to benefit from cross-pollination with swim training. I find that during the post-season, many athletes benefit from allowing run training to take more of a backseat in the training plan to truly allow muscular recovery and rejuvenation.

Case Study | The Running Trap

John is a solid Ironman competitor with plenty of racing experience, but he is frustrated by his run performance off the bike. Each season he has tried to improve his run performance but has been set back by a series of run-related injuries. Frustrated, he commits in the off-season to truly work on his running and enters a marathon. After spending the winter training for a spring marathon, he records a personal record (PR) and is excited for the Ironman season ahead.

John will likely finish the Ironman season with another disappointment. He is caught in an injury loop due to the fact that he plans too much load in his run training. John makes the mistake of thinking that his run performance is due to insufficient run training rather than looking for flaws in his swim and bike training or his preparation for race day. In spite of being an Ironman athlete, John has never established true consistency due to his injuries, and it's quite likely that he will not do so until he builds up the musculoskeletal platform to absorb the load that comes with running. Now John will go into the next season with muscular damage and fatigue from the marathon and either inadequate development of swimming or cycling or fatigue from maintaining swimming and cycling due to training for the marathon. Underlying all of this is the fact that running a marathon has little relation to running an Ironman marathon.

Triathletes need to give greater emphasis to specific run sessions. Rather than judging training by the duration of sessions or the number of miles accumulated in a week of training, focus should be placed on running with the best available form. Lots of running is needed, but lots of *good* running is critical. The question in this chapter is going to be how to develop a plan that provides the optimal load needed to evolve and also hits all the specific key sessions that will provide improvements without injury. Answering this question is, of course, both art and science, but it begins with the mind-set of the athlete and coach and their willingness to develop a truly patient and progressive program.

BENEFITS OF IMPROVED RUNNING

I don't think many would argue against improving in any of the three disciplines in the sport, but it is worth understanding how running improvements correlate with a ramp-up of overall performance and your development as an athlete. By truly evolving your running resilience and performance, you open many doors of opportunity to improve overall performance. These include:

Prevention of slowdown. The run is the discipline in which many triathletes experience their biggest slowdown, or poor performance relative to training levels. As the run occurs at the end of the race, this slowdown is not only due to run training or ability. Nonetheless, improving your running resilience, performance, and confidence will mean that you are less likely to crumble when things get tough.

Injury reduction. If being an improved runner leads to better musculoskeletal resilience, then such improvement will certainly lower the risk of injury.

I often see athletes who are consistently injured because they are simply not able to gain *enough* frequency or load in their training to develop the resilience necessary to absorb training. If you can develop the resilience, then you will not only improve but also be less likely to get injured. This dilemma shows why avoidance of injury eventually becomes more about smart training than about trying to build resilience.

Tactical development. Until you improve resilience and performance level, you are less able to develop a meaningful, thorough tactical and pacing strategy. For many, the run is about managing the slowdown, but evolving your performance will increase the opportunity to truly manage pacing, terrain, and interaction with your competitors.

Improved confidence. Athletes with a weaker run often race in fear and tend to sabotage any possible high-quality performance by working above their fitness and ability levels. Poor runners cannot help but aim to bank time because of the looming fear of a weak run split. You can easily see how this becomes a vicious cycle of failure and decreasing confidence. Improve the run, and you will reduce the desire to override your ability in your racing.

Ultimately, our sport is swim-bike-run. If you are successful in developing your swimming and riding, then the route to further performance gains is through the run. There is no point in setting up a great run performance with a smart and effective swim and bike if your running ability is limited.

RUNNING FORM

While some triathletes spend plenty of time seeking advice to magically improve their swimming form and will invest plenty of money in a proper bike fit, it seems that many are resistant to any real evolution of their running form. As with any of the disciplines, we could go into great depth on proper running biomechanics, but the complexity of the topic would probably leave most triathletes with little takeaway. Many brilliant running coaches and biomechanists who have great passion for running form may kick and scream over the simplicity of what I lay out, but I do so without apology. The fundamentals for improvement that I outline in this portion of the chapter will meet the needs of most triathletes. For my pro athletes, a discussion of proper running form will probably be a little different (although the basics remain the same), but what applies to them is more than the requirements and needs of most amateurs. So let's first focus on and improve the fundamentals and train for improvements; after that, you may explore the deeper or finer elements of form as you improve and evolve.

Posture

Proper running form begins with good posture: Stand tall to give yourself the best biomechanical advantage possible for deploying the finer elements of the sport. Similar to what we discussed in the swimming chapter, make your body taut, holding a straight line from chest to hips with your head in a neutral position. Ensure that you are not tucking your chin into your chest or letting your head fall back behind your shoulders. Great head position should be neutral, focused on the road about 25 to 35 feet in front of you.

Without losing that good, taut posture, you now want to tip forward from the ankles to ensure that your center of balance is just in front of neutral. You *do not bend from the waist*; instead, simply tilt (as if from the ankles) to kick-start the feeling of just barely falling forward. This is a subtle yet important cue to help gain consistent momentum in the run.

Troubleshooting Running Posture

Here are the most common mistakes runners make when it comes to posture.

- **Leading with the hips:** The shoulders fall behind the center line or hips, the head tips back, and the center of balance is behind neutral. This leads to loss of foot speed, deceleration, and a decrease in running economy.
- **Bending at the waist:** In an attempt to move the center of balance forward, the runner bends at the waist and the butt sticks out. Alignment is neutral rather than forward, and posture is poor.
- **Looking to the stars or the ground:** Posture is compromised by looking down at the feet or up at the sky.
- **Exaggerating the forward lean:** Too much lean will cause overrotation and increase the risk of injury due to the higher-impact force on landing.

Arm Carriage

I am a big fan of getting the arms "out of the way" for the majority of your running, then bringing them in for contribution to powering over hills or increasing overall speed or leg speed. Poor arm carriage can be disruptive to foot speed and running form, so ensuring that you carry the arms well will help your technique and assist in making your form more economical. Proper arm carriage begins with supple, relaxed shoulders and arms. Tuck the elbows behind the wrist so that the line from elbow to wrist is in line with the shoulder—that is, your forearm should not cross the midline of your body. Minimize forward swing—the only active portion of the arm carriage is a small drive back as the opposite knee moves forward. This swing action increases as you desire more foot speed or to drive up and over a hill or roller. The angle between the upper arm and the forearm is held at less than 90 degrees, as though you are holding a tennis ball between forearm and biceps.

Troubleshooting Arm Carriage

Following are the most common mistakes in arm carriage.

- **Crossing the midline:** The arm swing crosses the midline in front of the body with each step. This disrupts hip mobility and leads to biomechanical issues further down the chain.
- **Long arms:** The arms swing low, with the hands and wrists brushing the shorts. This typically leads to slower leg speed, a common issue for triathletes.
- **Overenthusiastic arms:** No one is seeking a nomination to the baton-twirling team, so avoid wild movements or swings. Keep the arms tidy and clean, conserving energy.

Hips

The hips are the power plant of good running form and performance. Too many athletes focus on driving through the back of the running stride, or where the foot is landing. Maintaining strong and stable hips can lead to maximum momentum, propulsion, and leg speed, which can lead to the biggest "aha!" moment for recreational runners. When fatigue sets in on the run,

FIGURE 8.1 : PROPER RUNNING FORM

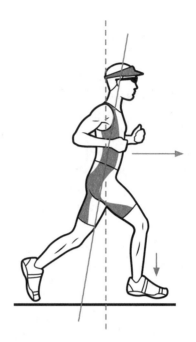

GOOD FORM
The athlete runs with tall posture and a center of balance (see gray line) that falls in front of the center line. The arm swing is compact, driving backward and then releasing the tension (not swinging forward). As the athlete drives his foot into the ground, creating potential energy, he is also moving forward. This means his foot will strike close to the center line.

many triathletes land on the foot and allow the hips to sink into the running stride, almost as if they are stuck in quicksand. This reduces the potential energy created by the landing because it loses energy into the ground; it also requires the runner to reverse deceleration and re-create acceleration, which takes time (with the foot on the ground) and massive energy. Here are some basic cues for stable, strong hips.

Keep the hips moving forward. When your foot lands, your aim should be to load and move the body and hips forward. This can be achieved only with proper posture and a subtle forward lean, but this mind-set will help load the landing leg and get propulsion initiated quickly. Keep the landing leg, led by the hips, strong and stable—the more you can do this, the greater the propulsive release as the body moves over the hips and springs off the back leg.

Raise the cadence. A result of loading the body and moving the hips forward is a likely, and welcome, improvement in leg speed. You cannot simply focus on leg speed for success, but maintaining foot speed, or cadence, is a key marker of running performance.

PROPULSION ON THE RUN: GETTING IT RIGHT

I find that most athletes achieve better form with a focus on strong hips instead of thinking about where or how the foot lands on the ground. That said, you will have problems if you are landing on tiptoe. This type of landing simply creates a break in momentum and takes away all biomechanical advantage of the design of the musculoskeletal system. It also radically increases load on the Achilles tendon and calf complex of muscles. It is an injury in waiting.

Furthermore, propulsion is driven by knee drive, not knee lift. We do want to get the knee forward quickly, from toe-off at the back of the stride to when the knee is at the highest point at the front of the stride, but don't lean back and simply lift the knee high, then let it passively fall toward the ground. Driving the leg into the ground is where you create your power and, if body position is great, propulsion and momentum. So stop playing "Knees Up, Mother Brown" (an old English song—look it up!).

Drive the leg into the ground. Strong, stable hips are a good stimulator to improve power. This has to be done with speed; hence it is no surprise that short, high-intensity hill repetitions are huge stimulators for improvements in form, economy, and running performance (even for Ironman athletes!).

Posture, arm carriage, and hips are fundamental to proper running form. Get these right and performance will follow because you will:

- Carry momentum forward with each stride, becoming a more economical runner
- Maintain foot speed, which is necessary for effective running off the bike
- Minimize negative impact forces that reduce speed or increase the injury risk or load on the musculoskeletal system

It is important to remember that, for most scenarios in triathlon, we are not actually running that fast relative to potential. Even the top Ironman athletes are running at a speed that is more focused on economy than on raw speed or maximal sustainable speed. Until you are focused on ITU professional

Olympic-distance racing or a few faster half-Ironman-distance races, the focus is on economy and remaining tidy and energy-efficient. Speed and intensity are critically important in training, but their purpose extends beyond simply increasing your maximal steady state.

The Effect of Fatigue on Running Form

Running is the discipline that suffers most when fatigue sets in. This is because we carry our full mass when we run, unlike swimming, where a great amount of weight is counteracted by the displacement of water. Furthermore, running forces us to create all of our own locomotion. When fatigue strikes, it is very challenging to maintain good form, and when form deteriorates, our sustainable speed drops. The overall cost of sustaining this now compromised form and speed goes up, and the vicious cycle continues. Symptoms of fatigue in running include:

Loss of Hip Stability	Failing to control hips, increasing lateral movement of the hips, and radically increasing the energy cost with each step
Weak Hips	Whether related to a weakened leg drive (from high knee into ground), lazy hip movement, or poor body position, we tend to see the hips sinking into the ground with each foot strike. This creates a lag in foot speed, a large deceleration in each step, and a need to re-create momentum with each step.
Passive Body Position	As fatigue sets in, athletes have a tendency to sit back, losing momentum. This slows leg speed, increases the cost of each foot strike, and extends the time that the foot remains on the ground.
Increased Neurological Cost	Form becomes very untidy with fatigue, compromising the ability to synchronize movement. The brain has a harder time communicating with the muscles, and more supporting or auxiliary muscles are enlisted in an effort to maintain form. Once again, cost is driven up, further adding to overall fatigue.

It's not hard to see how all of these symptoms are related. There is not one specific area that is solely responsible for your decline. They all add up and contribute to the fatigue equation.

TRAINING THE RUN IN TRIATHLON

Beyond simply getting faster, the goal of run training is to create a sustainable program that will ensure that you remain injury-free while also improving your speed and endurance, both cardiovascular and muscular. When reviewing many athletes' running programs, I often see a paradoxical situation in a plan that only has them running two to three times weekly, but with each session carrying so much load, or creating so much stress, that the fatigue consequences are great. When this "big" running approach is combined with the essential swimming and biking, the result is a consistently accumulating recipe of fatigue and muscle damage, leading to little performance gains or even injury. Ironically, many make their biggest mistake before the season has begun, with the noble aim of creating a running base or foundation.

The common approach is to accumulate very easy extended miles of longer running sessions throughout the winter months with the aim of creating a platform of fitness that can sustain the tougher sessions later in the year. This idea is all very well, but it misses a key point of running progression. As mentioned previously, we have to consider not only the cardiovascular stress of run training but also the musculoskeletal stress. Running is weight-bearing and produces great muscular damage. The less efficient the runner, the greater the muscular damage. If we compare a human body to a car, the muscles, bones, ligaments, and tendons are the chassis. This chassis can be strengthened through careful progressive training and can be developed to absorb great training load. Unfortunately, long and easy winter miles are the worst possible method of developing musculoskeletal resilience because the load is typically too great for the athlete to absorb and respond to.

It is critical to understand that infrequent long runs cannot prepare the body for greater load. Keep this concept in the front of your mind when focusing on running progression. If you want to learn how to play the guitar, you shouldn't just pick it up and spend several hours strumming on the weekend. Setting aside a little time daily to practice would be a better approach. Try a similar approach with your run training. The only safe route is frequent, shorter runs. This concept acts as the platform to *start* our planning of run training within triathlon. Of course, to accept and follow this progression takes massive patience, a little planning, and a touch of vision. It's not easy for the ambitious and highly motivated athlete, but those who follow this path usually come out on top. We follow this premise in setting up the season of run training.

Setting Up Your Year

The progression of run training over a season looks something like this: Build the chassis, work on endurance and strength progression, sharpen, and then transition to training for the specifics of your race. Rinse and repeat, season after season.

Post-season Run Training

Reduced training stress
Emphasis on technique and skills
Frequency over duration

Focus on preparing the body for the heavy training load ahead. There is more freedom to keep intensity light and sessions short to create strong musculoskeletal resilience.

Following a post-racing break, we are now ready to begin ramping up for the next season. Don't worry; the hard work is still some way off! The initial goal of the season is to *prepare the body for run training.* While this goal does involve training, view it as preparation—this will prevent you from going too fast or doing too much too soon. The simple mission of the post-season phase is to build musculoskeletal resilience, establish good running form (or focus on improving baseline running form), and gradually increase cardiovascular fitness. You will notice that there are little to no long durations. *The goal is for frequency of running to progress, which means we will avoid sessions that cause massive fatigue or muscular damage.*

This phase of training will typically last 8 to 10 weeks and occur in October through the New Year (for Northern Hemisphere athletes). *Frequency, form, and freedom from fatigue* is your mantra. So how much frequency is appropriate, and how is it integrated into the week? Well, I am afraid the answer is "It depends," but there are some guidelines to help you figure it out.

Because most athletes will be focused on swimming, combined with functional strength and riding progression, at this part of the season, think of sneaking in short run sessions throughout the week. For example, I like to have athletes split their running into two shorter sessions within a day, which may accumulate a reasonable daily mileage but without as much risk of damage or significant fatigue. For more established athletes, or those with a great amount of free time, this might mean progressing to the point that you are fitting in

EASING OFF THE RUN IN THE POST-SEASON

After a long season of training and racing, nearly all athletes benefit from an extended period in which consistent run training takes a backseat to allow full muscular healing and repair. For most athletes, it takes two to three weeks to effectively "reset" the body for another season. It will feel as if you are going backward in terms of fitness, but the rejuvenation will work wonders for your consistency in the coming season. During this time, feel free to remain active with unstructured training. If you do choose to run, the runs should be very short and social—no intervals. I prefer a couple of weeks of real relaxation and an emotional and physical break from anything resembling triathlon progression. The key to making this approach pay off is to take great caution as you return to your training progression.

The idea of easing off run training is particularly challenging if you view yourself as an accomplished runner. After all, your strongest discipline is your safe zone, in which you feel free, strong, and confident. To place it on the back burner is a challenge to your ego, confidence, and even enjoyment of the sport. Backing away from significant volume or intensity for a few weeks at the end of the season allows true healing to occur while also opening the opportunity to build winter fitness and progression in the all-important swimming portion of the sport. If you *begin* with a healing phase and then progress to construction of a platform of resilience that you can continue to build from, your chances of injury decrease, and performance gains from the hard running ahead will be greater. This does not mean you cannot run in the post-season, but any running you do should not be in pursuit of working on the run or improving run speed.

7 to 10 running sessions in each week. That sounds daunting, but none of the sessions should last longer than 50 minutes and most will be 20 to 40 minutes, so the total accumulation of load is not great. For the more typical athlete who is also juggling family, work, and a busy life, this run progression may get you up to 5 to 7 runs weekly with similar durations for each session (or even less). Not all of these runs should be stand-alone sessions—many can effectively and efficiently be coupled with other sessions. For instance, they may precede or follow a functional strength session or a swim. Nearly all of these running

sessions can be very low intensity, but form and technical improvements are the backbone of each session.

We aim to place great focus on the main elements of running technique, and the only intervals or structure imbedded in these sessions are designed to improve the dialogue between your brain and running muscles. Form-based, higher-intensity strides and hill work, as well as some potential drills, support the motor programming that occurs from increasing frequency with shorter duration. Beyond resilience, we gain improvements in running gait through forcing the brain to connect with the running muscles with great consistency. This approach reiterates the point that more is not better. It heightens the focus and the demand to *not* run with fatigue at this stage of the season. This is the critical point that determines how much, how often, and how long. You will need to make logical decisions about your progression and avoid the desire for more or instant gratification in your running progression.

FORM-BASED POWER INTERVALS

This session includes some higher intensity, but it's designed to trigger neuro-muscular recruitment of running muscles and improve power potential without residual fatigue. The key is complete recovery between the hill intervals.

Warm-up	**5 min.** easy walking into
	5 min. dynamic warm-up exercises
Pre–Main Set	**10–20 min.** low-stress running, Z2
	Take walk breaks as needed to maintain form.
Main Set	**6 to 8 × 30–40 sec.** at Z5 on a grade of 4–7%
	Walk downhill for 2 min. rest between each interval.
	Run with high power and great form: focus on posture, lean, arm carriage, and power potential, with knee driving into the ground while retaining stable hips.
	5–10 min. easy running Z2 with great form to finish

Note: *Find options for dynamic warm-up exercises in Appendix B.*

LOW-STRESS ENDURANCE RUN

Beautiful in its simplicity, this is a typical session for this part of the season. Notice the shorter duration and the lack of intervals as well as the walk breaks to limit stress and injury risk. These measures allow for optimal form. We are not chasing big fitness yet.

Warm-up	**5 min.** easy walking into
	5 min. dynamic warm-up exercises
Main Set	**30–50 min.** Z2, with 20–30 sec. walking every sixth minute
	Every third and sixth minute, focus on posture, body position, and foot speed to retain proper form.

Note: *Find options for dynamic warm-up exercises in Appendix B.*

Pre-season Run Training

Gradually improve cardiovascular and muscular endurance
Retain form and skills focus
Introduce real power intervals for form and technical development

Ensure that you keep the easy running very easy. Running at a moderately strong effort at this phase of the season will cause fatigue and may heighten your risk of injury.

If you have followed a careful progression of running frequency, you should move into the new year with a sound foundation of musculoskeletal integrity and almost no residual fatigue from the run training already completed. You may also be well on the way to technical improvements, especially if your run training has been a low-stress habit rather than an anchor of your weekly training week. So this must be the time to pile on the miles and begin building that massive foundation, right? I am afraid not. You are going to have to give up on the notion of long, slow distance and traditional base-building running—it has no place in triathlon running progression. This is why a winter marathon is the wrong approach!

The focus of the pre-season is to gradually transition the emphasis from pure musculoskeletal resilience, cardiovascular endurance, and form and to begin increasing overall load. The theme remains *frequency over single-session duration* in the vast majority of sessions, but the specificity and duration of two to three foundational, or key, sessions each week will begin to progress. Don't forget that many athletes will still be focusing on swimming, riding, and functional strength as their primary disciplines in this phase, but we do get to increase run load. The likelihood is that we will maintain the run frequency, and if you are at a high number of runs weekly, most will remain similar in focus, with easy intensity and short duration. The transition occurs in the key sessions, with two to three sessions progressing to that point. The first will be a focus on form-based power, with a session focused on improving the pure recruitment and power potential of running form. This typically involves hill-based running, with efforts that are short in duration (30 to 60 seconds) and at high intensity. Complete recovery occurs between each, as the focus is on recruitment and power, not general fitness. While intensity is very high, the total amount of work in these sessions is very low, and the resulting fatigue is also low. I find that athletes get frustrated with these sessions because they fail to provide the "give-back" buzz of a tough interval session or long run, but their value is high.

The second session of the week is a progression of pure endurance within a session—or, put another way, an increase in duration. This medium-endurance run places stress on you by extending duration, but the goal is still good form. This means there needs to be a careful progression of duration over the entire pre-season phase. I will often combine this session with an element of strength by requesting that it be completed on hilly or rolling terrain, but it is important to remember that hills and rolling terrain must still be navigated with good form. More established runners, or those with more time to train, may include a third key session that is a pure strength-based session. Often completed on the treadmill at medium intensity and relatively shallow grade (3 to 5 percent), this low-stress and form-based strength session includes short to medium-length intervals to assist in recruitment and endurance. Don't mistake these sessions for traditional hill repetitions, which conjure images of standing at the top of the hill, bent over at the waist following another gut-wrenching effort to summit. We don't go there yet!

As this two- to three-month phase progresses, we will begin to increase the length of the medium-duration run and place a heavier emphasis on the strength-based element of running. Your form and resilience should improve, and capacity to absorb running load should become greater. As you progress toward the end of this phase, you should become what I call a balanced triathlete. Your swimming, biking, and running will have a more traditionally balanced load within the week, although this doesn't mean balanced total training hours in each discipline.

Thinking of your run training as becoming balanced only after months of lower focus leads many to assume that running becomes exposed as an area of weakness. This simply isn't true. The truth is that we have been *very* focused on run progression throughout the last months, but the backseat approach of overall training load is exactly what has been necessary to progress running resilience, form, and fitness while allowing you to also develop as a triathlete overall. Remember, we aim to become best at swim-bike-run, not swimming, biking, and running. The sports are not mutually exclusive. If you have the courage to follow this very careful progression throughout post-season and pre-season, you will have sneakily built great resilience, improved your form, and become more fit than you realize. You should be in a great place to take on the more demanding load that comes next.

FORM-BASED POWER INTERVALS

We progress from the teaser power of the last block and introduce higher-intensity and -load intervals. The focus is endurance and form progression, and this session fits within this equation despite the presence of intensity.

Warm-up	**5 min.** easy walking into
	5 min. dynamic warm-up exercises
Pre–Main Set	**10–20 min.** low-stress running, Z2
	Walk as needed to maintain form.
Main Set	**8 to 12 × up to 1 min.** Z5 with great form
	Rest 3 min. between each interval.
	These intervals are very strong, but proper posture, arm carriage, body position, and foot speed are a must. This will challenge you. As soon as form declines, stop that interval.
	Full recovery is critical to be effective in the main set.

Note: *Find options for dynamic warm-up exercises in Appendix B.*

EXTENDED ENDURANCE INTERVALS

While most of the supporting sessions will be at or under 50 minutes of total duration, you do get to embrace an occasional extended endurance session. Executing good form and limiting damage remain the primary goals.

Warm-up	**5 min.** easy walking into
	5 min. dynamic warm-up exercises
Main Set	**70–90 min.** low-stress running, Z2
	Walk as needed to maintain form—typically 30 sec. every sixth minute.
	Every third minute, focus on form.
	You can use a metronome, or Tempo Trainer, to maintain foot speed with the goal of running easy with great form and foot speed. Set the Tempo Trainer 2 to 5 steps per minute faster than your regular foot speed.

Note: *Find options for dynamic warm-up exercises in Appendix B.*

Sustainable Power Run Training

Great diversity in intensity, from easy sessions to higher-intensity sessions
Form over fight—never compromise supple and relaxed form

A proper warm-up, as well as postexercise fueling, is the best way to limit damage from the higher-intensity running sessions and allows optimal recovery. Don't skip your easy warm-up.

I prefer the focus for this phase to be on sharpening, but sustainable power has become common lore in purplepatch training, so I'll keep it here. Often coupled with the commencement of early-season racing, an emphasis on sustainable power marks an increase of overall intensity of the running load and a real divergence of intensity between the sessions in a given week, or block, of training. Your early-season races will often take the place of some of the key sessions in this phase and assist in the great increase of muscular endurance and resilience at race intensity. We are beginning to prepare to become able to sustain racing intensity; hence an increase of focus in sustained intensity and speed is appropriate. Most athletes will quickly learn that with a couple of more intense and demanding sessions within the training plan, supporting runs will need to become even lighter and easier. Some athletes will even need to drop the frequency of runs within the week of training to allow appropriate recovery from the tougher sessions.

One of the key sessions of each block will include a more traditional session with track or hill repetitions. Working on maximal sustainable effort and speed, these form-based interval sessions resemble classical run training for most athletes. With the combined load of cycling and swimming, it is doubtful that you would include both hard hill work and sustained flat interval work within a single week, but both have their place in the training fabric.

These maximal-effort sessions are balanced with a focus on increasing the duration at which you can hold tempo pace. It requires real focus to hold form while operating at a moderately high, suffocation-inducing pace. Think of tempo running as *hard but not breathless, often in the upper area of Z3 or up to the middle of Z4.* These sessions are great venues for learning how to maintain form while in discomfort and are massive stimulators of endurance and sustainable speed. The key is to avoid going *too hard* in them; failure should never be allowed to occur in a single session.

The final area of intensity within a week of training in this phase might come in the form of the more traditional run following a bike session, often referred to as a "brick." This skills-based session has a place in this phase of training because it is so specific to the sport. To achieve the desired effect, a brick run should be at or above race intensity and short in duration. Early in the year, I usually ask for a building effort or speed to allow the dialogue between brain and muscles to occur naturally, but this means that we do hit some higher intensity in the final portion of the short run.

Throughout this phase, only the most accomplished runners will be able to maintain the one or two medium-endurance sessions that were part of the pre-season progression. Less-established athletes need to focus on shorter, low-intensity supporting runs to maintain endurance. While I highlight the shift in intensity in this phase, don't mistake it for a classic power-and-speed phase of traditional periodization. The focus is not solely on improving power and speed, so don't reduce training volume to achieve the goals established. Instead, facilitate a natural progression of load balanced with increasing intensity within the week of run training. Up to this point in the season, we have been building strength, resilience, endurance, and form. While the fundamentals of running performance have been established, you are not yet race-ready. This *sustained power* phase acts as the natural sharpening transition toward race-readiness and performance evolution. Think of it as a shift in mind-set and focus but not a harsh deviation from your natural progression. If you have been smart and patient, resisting the urge to load up with fatigue-inducing long, slow runs early in the season, this is where it pays off. You will really begin to feel fit, strong, and more powerful in your running. You will likely have some good experiences in your early-season races, with the promise of even better things to come.

BEST SUSTAINED EFFORT INTERVALS

We progress from the teaser power of the last block to introduce higher-intensity and -load intervals. The focus is endurance and form progression, and this session fits within this equation despite the presence of intensity.

Warm-up	**5 min.** easy walking into
	5 min. dynamic warm-up exercises
Pre–Main Set 1	**10–15 min.** low-stress running, Z2
	Walk as needed to maintain form.
Pre–Main Set 2	**3 to 5 × 90 sec.** Ramp effort by 30 sec. to Z3/4, walk 30 sec. between intervals.
Main Set	**8 × 4–7 min.**
	Progress the effort over first 4 intervals to very strong and sustainable effort. Then maintain that pace for the last 4 intervals.
	Always allow 4–7 min. complete rest between each interval (match recovery to interval duration).

Note: Find options for dynamic warm-up exercises in Appendix B.

HILLY ENDURANCE SPLIT RUN

The focus of the phase is best sustained power, but that doesn't mean we hit every key session with high-intensity intervals because that would simply create fatigue and injury risk. We still want to improve muscular endurance throughout this phase. To reduce muscular damage, split your run into multiple sessions throughout the day. You will see the "option" component here, depending on how you are feeling.

A.M. Run

Warm-up	**5 min.** easy walking into
	5 min. dynamic warm-up exercises
Main Set	**30–45 min.** Z2 smooth endurance run
	Walk breaks if needed

P.M. Run

Warm-up	**5 min.** easy walking into
	5 min. dynamic warm-up exercises
Main Set	**40–70 min.** hilly endurance
	If your legs are heavy and fatigued, simply maintain form and Z2 throughout. Walk the steeper grades. If your legs feel fresh and vibrant, progress from easy endurance to strong and sustained.
	Don't be limited by zones today.

Note: *Find options for dynamic warm-up exercises in Appendix B.*

Race-Specific Run Training

Until this point we have focused on developing you as a runner, with improved resilience, form, endurance, power, and sustainable speed. We now need to focus specifically on your key events. Similar to what we mapped out for the cycling program, later-season Ironman races may have a progression of focus within this long season, with the goal of improving half-Ironman performance earlier in the racing season, then progressing to the greater load of Ironman training in the 9 to 13 weeks prior to race day. This phase of training has a greater emphasis on race-specific intensity, pacing sessions, and skills-based run sessions that occur immediately following bike sessions in brick workouts.

Whether preparing for short-course sprint and Olympic distances or the challenge of Ironman, remember that you will still include the full range of intensities within each week, or block, of training. Short-course training doesn't mean all running sessions are at race pace, in the same way that Ironman training is not focused on long-duration and low-intensity running. The key difference is that the *focus* and *amount* of intensity vary dramatically.

For the short-course athlete, the key sessions are the heart of the training week and are mostly focused on improving the highest sustainable pace as well as acting as dress rehearsals for race-specific demands. Because the intensity of short-course racing is much higher than that of long-course racing, the intensity of these key sessions is relatively high. This means that nearly all additional running within a week, or block, is designed as either recovery, simple endurance maintenance, or preparation for another upcoming key session. For all of these supporting sessions, the intensity will be much lower, but they do play an important role in maintaining resilience and endurance. It is worth pointing out that these supporting sessions are often the ones that cause problems, not because of their inclusion but because of poor execution on the athlete's part. It is very common for athletes to run supporting sessions at too high an intensity, instantly shifting their nature and load. It is tough for any coach to persuade a highly motivated athlete of the value of lower-intensity running as these sessions fail to build confidence or boost the ego. This is why it is key to understand the value and the purpose of each session and why a good coach will never say, "Because I said so," when asked why the session is included in the week!

The emphasis for the long-course athlete will be on improving the form and speed over extended-duration sessions and programming the body to become fine-tuned and highly efficient at a pace that is relatively low when compared to the athlete's maximal sustainable speed. The stress comes from the duration of the session, whether it is in extended intervals or simply longer-duration running, but the overall intensity is low. While supporting runs still have a role in recovery from and preparation for key sessions, I like to include higher intensity in some of the supporting sessions to maintain neurological firing, form improvements, and muscular recruitment. A touch of speed work is all that is necessary to prevent athletes from becoming single-speed "diesel-engine" runners and to maintain the benefits established earlier in the season.

OLYMPIC-DISTANCE-SPECIFIC RUN

Form always supersedes fight, so retain great form
Higher-intensity intervals are not necessarily at your best effort
Be cautious in how often you hit very high intensity each week

If it is challenging to hit a key running interval session in the week, we will typically add a race-specific brick run on the back of a higher-intensity bike interval session. This will be a shorter session that forces race-specific speed.

The typical amateur triathlete can run at the prescribed pace—that is, over race pace. The feeling should be "very strong but sustainable," so I avoid calling it a "best effort" or "maximal effort." That is not specific. For more elite athletes, the pace might be closer to specific goal race pace.

Warm-up	**5 min.** easy walking into
	5 min. dynamic warm-up exercises
Pre–Main Set	**15 min.** Z2
	In every third minute, build effort by 20 sec. to very strong and flowing Z4 running in the last 20 sec.
Main Set	**8 to 12 × 4 min.** at 105% of race goal pace
	Run easy for 4 min. between intervals
	As soon as you fail to maintain the pace, drop the interval by 30 sec.
	If you fail to retain at least 3 minutes at this speed, you are either too tired to perform the workout properly or have an overly ambitious race-pace goal!

Note: *Find options for dynamic warm-up exercises in Appendix B.*

HALF-IRONMAN-SPECIFIC RUN

Half-Ironman race pace is not best effort
Practice taking in fuel during the intervals, not the breaks
Efforts are controlled with good form

Many athletes run too fast in the half-Ironman-specific sessions. Retain some speed work, but use this session as a dress rehearsal. In other words, don't run these intervals at your stand-alone 5K or 10K pace!

The main goal is to fine-tune extended intervals to be at, or just above, your race-pace effort. You should only complete intervals in which you can maintain good form and the required intensity.

| Warm-up | **5 min.** easy walking into |
| | **5 min.** dynamic warm-up exercises |

Pre–Main Set	**15–20 min.**, build every one-third to Z3/3+ in the final third. Walk 2–3 min.
Main Set	**2 to 5 × 12–18 min.** at sustained Z3+ effort *Focus on great posture, leg speed, and body position.*

Note: *Find options for dynamic warm-up exercises in Appendix B.*

IRONMAN-SPECIFIC RUN

Ironman running involves strength and endurance, not speed
We are deep into specificity now—key sessions are dress rehearsals for races
Some speed work is still valuable

Remember to keep the easy very easy and that Ironman race speed is not very fast relative to your best sustainable speed. Ironman-specific runs should not be tests of speed but tests of patient and proper execution.

We place the intervals at the end of the run, as this is where the endurance-based focus needs to occur, and also because it encourages proper pacing on race day. Feel free to keep the early part of this run very easy.

Warm-up	**5 min.** easy walking into **5 min.** dynamic warm-up exercises
Pre–Main Set	**45–60 min.** very-low-stress running, Z1/2 Take walk breaks to maintain form.
Main Set	**3 × 20 min.** as 5 min. easier than Ironman race pace, 10 min. at race pace, 5 min. just faster than race pace Walk 2 min. between each interval.

Note: *Find options for dynamic warm-up exercises in Appendix B.*

part III

TURNING POTENTIAL INTO PERFORMANCE

9

Mapping Your Path to Performance

I am often surprised by how many athletes end up deploying a "rinse and repeat" strategy when it comes to training and race progression. They go through a season like a pinball, bouncing from race to race and simply training for the demands of that next upcoming event. At the end of the season, they might take a little break; then it is right back to the next season. Now, there is little wrong with this approach if your goal is to enjoy the sport, have fun in competing, and ensure that you get a health benefit from the training and racing, but it is not the route to ongoing positive results and performance. Unfortunately, you *have* to tailor your plan to achieve real progression as an athlete.

Even newer athletes or those with modest ambitions benefit from employing a longer-term view of their sport and progression. Why? The biggest reason is that true development and great improvement can seldom be created in just a few months or a single season. Each year of training and racing should build on the last one, allowing continual evolution and improvements and resulting in greater and greater performance levels. If this is the case, it is best to plan for that and to frame our seasons and events within this context.

You need to create a road map toward becoming a better athlete and use it as a guide to build a season of training and racing. Bear in mind that early-season races have to be slotted into the progression of training, but they shouldn't dictate the training. The progression is the priority; after it is established, then such events may be added without impeding the overall plan (unlike key races, which require specific preparation). Progressive training is the key to forcing adaptations and improvement. Now that we have addressed how to achieve it within each individual sport, you can combine it with the wisdom and lessons learned from racing, and you will be on your way to success.

GOAL SETTING: ASK THE RIGHT QUESTIONS

Where would you like to be in three years? This is the most important question I ask my athletes. The best way to approach such a big question is to imagine yourself in three years' time and think of scenarios that would make you happy. (Of course it doesn't *have* to be three years; it can be slightly less or more.) What outcomes excite you? Even if it feels a little out of reach, a goal that elicits this kind of positive anticipation can provide the direction you need. Most talk about goal-setting stresses the need to set goals that are objective and measurable, but I believe you can take a more relaxed approach for this long-range plan. Although you will need to approach the coming year with very specific goals, your overarching vision for the years that will follow can be your guiding light for the path ahead. Ensure that you create a vision and then a concrete plan for how you will make it a reality.

The logistics of mapping a season are complicated by the fact that participation in triathlon is growing. The most popular races are in high demand, forcing athletes to commit to race entries up to a year in advance. When the big races sell out, many are forced to choose different races. Although obstacles like this are not ideal, my hope is that you are able to take a step back and map a smart progression for your season. It is critical to remember that you cannot be firing on all cylinders throughout an entire season. There are typically a couple of periods within a calendar year in which you can aim to be at your best conditioning and readiness for performance. Your key races should be planned accordingly, with specific preparation in the buildup to race day. Don't despair; this doesn't mean that racing occurs only in short phases and the rest of the season is a wash. Breakthroughs and stellar race results can be attained outside these "performance windows," but the nature of progressive training that can elicit real gains is that it prepares an athlete to be truly race-ready in a relatively small portion of the season. For athletes in the Northern

Hemisphere, the race-specific phase of training sprawls from May through October or November. Within this phase of racing, you can likely afford to build toward key races a couple of times. This usually entails a peak phase in May, June, or July and another peak in October or November. Of course this is a gross generalization because the timing also depends on the individual athlete, but it provides some context for your mapping and planning.

I encourage athletes to think of their season as two miniseasons. After the first goal race or series of races, we include a break lasting 7 to 21 days to allow physical and emotional recuperation. This break is not as deep as the one at the end of the season. A short break with continued activity, albeit at a lower stress level, allows a little healing and a mental break from the grind. With recovery taken care of, the second half of the season can be approached with vigor, allaying fears of becoming stale or accumulating too much fatigue.

When you map your key events and training for those events, *consider where you need to be by the end of the season* to set up your progression toward the longer-term dream or vision. Some give-and-take might be necessary in the short term to make this progression happen. Many athletes chase bigger results in their current season, thus jeopardizing their ultimate dream. I recently began coaching a very talented triathlete with a weakness in swimming. His approach to training has been very balanced, with three swimming sessions each week. For him to truly evolve as a pro and succeed at that level, his swim must improve. We are planning a weighted emphasis on swimming this season to set him up to handle and absorb the heavy swim load in the season that follows. His swim progression will be a multiyear journey, so year one needs to be organized with the coming couple of years in mind.

STAGING RACES

Here lies the key mistake that many athletes make when framing the season. Not all races are created equal. While you should race each race to the best of your ability, you don't need to be primed for every race in your season. As mentioned earlier, true peak fitness and performance ability can be maintained for only a few weeks and should be targeted only a couple of times within each season. That said, most triathletes like to race—and should race! If you have mapped your season to provide optimal readiness in the summer and early-fall months, early-season races that occur in March, April, and even May should be viewed through a very different lens than those in July or October. More than stepping stones to the main events, early-season races (or B races) are great benchmarks of fitness, can be good test runs for strategy and fueling, and provide valuable feedback on progression to athlete and coach. B races don't require the same emotional weight or physical preparation as A races, and they should not distract from the main focus of training and preparation. Having clear A and B designations can release you from the internal pressure of wanting the best possible performance in every single event. A word of warning: While you may designate an early-season race as a B race, or whatever tag suits you, such priority-setting doesn't mean it's acceptable to approach it with a lackadaisical attitude. I like athletes to race every time they toe the line. You want to put forth your best effort, be open to a wonderful performance, and ensure that the process and outcome of the event provide a chance for learning and assessment. I have had athletes of all levels perform very well in early-season racing, but our hope is that their performances in these early races will be eclipsed by performances later in the season.

To cement this thought process, think about your season by initially focusing on the process of training, then evolving toward the focus on racing as you progress. Early-season races fall into the progression of training, but race-readiness for your key races is the top priority for all key training sessions you hope to achieve. This is why many say it is better to arrive at a race 10 percent less fit than 1 percent overcooked. The goal is to reach the start fit, healthy, and prepared to race.

Case Study | The Route to Kona Qualification

Terry dreams of qualifying for the sport's holy grail, the Hawaii Ironman World Championships. By this point in his triathlon career, he has completed a few Ironman races, but he has failed to put together a balanced and strong Ironman event. Terry sees himself as a weaker swimmer, a relatively solid biker, and a talented runner. He feels that he lacks power on the bike because he struggles to ride at a much faster pace in half-Ironman distances than in Ironman, and he has trouble with running off the bike.

Path to Performance

Terry needs to carefully consider which race he will target. He needs to consider his history of qualifications, the race course and profile, typical environmental conditions, and other contributing factors. He then needs to weigh these factors against his strengths and weaknesses. If he is terrible in hot conditions or unable to capitalize on flatter courses, he should avoid selecting a flat, hot course!

Before race day, Terry needs to *evolve as an athlete*. He is not yet ready to race at the level that would typically merit qualification. To begin the evolution, he needs to improve swim performance, sustainable power on the bike, and running off the bike. Without targeting these three areas, Terry might see incremental improvements, but they are not likely to be enough. Here is a look at how this could play out for Terry.

Evolve the athlete. Terry will likely need one or two seasons to raise the ceiling of his performance. This is more easily done at the shorter-distance events, so he should stage the first half of the coming season or two with the goal of improving sustainable power and half-Ironman performance.

Swim project. Terry will dedicate himself to swim evolution, beginning a two-year project with heavy emphasis in the winter months. The emphasis on swim training will extend throughout the season, supported by participation in a competitive environment to raise swim performance.

Ironman racing. Because Terry has experienced poor running off the bike in multiple races, I would stage all Ironman races in the latter part of the season so as not to interrupt the goal of improving half-Ironman performance. I believe positive experiences provide the best learning. Throughout the season, Terry should focus on running well. This may require a more conservative riding approach, especially with his newfound power from early-season training. A more conservative approach to riding will open the opportunity to run well, and this can be a platform for growth and confidence.

If all goes well, Terry will arrive at the end of the first or second season with an improved swim (and the lessons he takes out of that journey), improved bike prowess, and confidence that he can run strong off the bike. He will also have a nagging feeling that the previous Ironman race or races went well, but there is much more in the bank now. After the first full season, he will be ready to build a season with one or two opportunities to race an Ironman at a new level, with a more balanced approach and closer to the level required for qualification.

While this all sounds logical and easy, most athletes don't have the patience to build the road map and stick to it. Most simply chase Ironman race after Ironman race with the goal of qualification. Too often, the 11.5-hour Ironman athlete is three years down the road and only 15 minutes faster.

TIP

Recognize that if you are like most athletes, qualification requires multiple seasons of progression and training. If you are willing to take on a goal that extends past a single season, your results are likely to reflect the time invested.

THE SECRET TO PERFORMANCE

When it comes down to the details of endurance training, every athlete wants to know what it will take to achieve success. Many triathletes are on a mission to find the secret sauce, or magic recipe, that prominent coaches use to create performance. I'm often asked about the types of intervals I create for my athletes, the number of hours of training I prescribe, and how long it takes to get results. The most popular questions from athletes seeking big performance gains are:

- How many hours a week do I have to train?
- How long do I need to get ready for X?

The frustrating response must be "I don't know." Questions like these tell me a lot about the athletes. To successfully coach them, I will need to educate them in how best to approach the sport, recalibrate their notions of how much they need to train, and convince them to take a broader view of performance gains.

A successful plan for endurance performance will take into account more than just an athlete's current level of fitness and the amount of time available for training. You must be willing to apply a dynamic and moving strategy to create effective training. There are certainly some traits shared by the most successful athletes, but simply emulating the pros is not a winning strategy. Throughout this chapter I will make some distinctions between the professional and the working amateur triathlete who seeks performance within the context of a busy life. I will outline the differences and similarities in hopes of helping you recognize the limiters and advantages that should be factored into your own training plan. If there is a secret to be discovered, it's self-awareness.

The Professional Athlete

These athletes are the icons of our sport, and their performance inspires all of us to be better, but simply emulating their approach to training or racing is a dangerous approach. We will explore many of the lessons to be learned from elite athletes, but suffice it to say, their lives and approach are very different from yours.

Quite simply, a professional's goal is to develop into a world-class athlete, winning races and championships. Everything is based on elite performance. This is important because some of the decisions made and approaches utilized may be at the expense of a full and complete life. While competing at the top or making the journey toward it, pros must have a myopic lens on maximizing performance. Not much else matters. Of course athletes are not robots, so smart coaches and athletes will do all that they can to round out this narrowly focused life with just enough real-life balance to ensure that passion and enjoyment are maintained—but I think you get the concept. Following are the ways that the professional triathlete goes about achieving this goal.

Minimize Life Stress

To maximize the body's absorption of specific training stress, the pro must radically reduce sources of life stress that cause negative hormonal stress. This means that any work outside training must be minimal; obligations to sponsors and organizations should be carefully managed; and absolute focus and value should be placed on sleep, rest, recuperation, and proper nutrition. The global goal is to create a comfortable setting with minimal life stress, leaving greater capacity for training.

One of the greatest stressors is a lack of supporting finances and sponsors. It's not an easy problem to solve, but it certainly factors into training ability for developing pro athletes. Many coaches see a rise in training and racing performance once an athlete manages to create a comfortable environment with reduced financial or sponsorship stress.

Maximize Training Load

The pro's training goal is to absolutely maximize training load while remaining in a state of positive adaptation. More *is* more, but only if the athlete is able to absorb and adapt to the stimulus. To determine *how much* training is enough, the athlete must take into account experience, individual resilience, and injury history and risk.

Experience. Training history and the foundation of fitness affect the athlete's capacity to absorb training. It takes time to develop the bedrock of fitness to successfully achieve greater load.

Individual resilience. Each athlete tends to have a predisposition for different types of training load. Some athletes respond better to lower intensity, whereas others are able to achieve a higher training load without consequences. These are also the athletes who tend to recuperate and bounce back from heavy sessions more quickly. Ironically, the fragile athlete is sometimes easier for a coach to manage and guide because the deeply resilient athlete can mask fatigue and initial stages of injuries for an extended time, which can lead to more serious issues.

Injury history and risk. Some athletes are bound by their history of injury, whether due to impact or overuse, and they have to carefully manage their training load in order to stay healthy. Because triathlon comprises three sports, if a previous injury in one of the sports requires management, athletes can often make up for it in another discipline.

The Amateur Athlete

The amateur must find a sustainable recipe of training that is in balance with the other factors in his or her life. This is where things get interesting. In the perfect scenario, all of the training becomes habitual within an already full and enriching life. In a sport as complex and demanding as triathlon, this scenario isn't easy to achieve, but it is a worthwhile pursuit. Unless you are a young amateur with aspirations to develop into the pro ranks, you should resist the temptation to allow the sport to dominate most or all of your bucket of life.

The vast majority of successful long-term triathletes should strive to maintain a full and happy life that can sustain training and racing while improving performance. Of course there are also goals of podium finishes, qualifications for championship events, personal records, and other performance markers, but all of these should be balanced with other elements of a complete life.

Balance Life Stress and Training Stress

A balanced life facilitates performance gains, so the goal is to integrate training into the framework of life. This immediately creates the need to consider each of the other factors in our lives that will minimize our ability to effectively

TRAINING TIME: WHEN LESS IS BEST

A relatively high-performing amateur came to me frustrated by a lack of performance gains. With multiple Hawaii Ironmans under the belt, he had plenty of experience. In order to review his downward trend, I had to go back more than five years, to the point where he had been given a big promotion at work. Over the five years that followed, the demands of his job had skyrocketed, with increased pressure and hours to work. He had failed to account for this in his approach to training. Rather than adjusting the approach and hours, he had aimed to maintain the same training program he had used before the promotion and simply set the alarm an extra hour early each weekday morning. Eventually the 6 a.m. alarm became 4 a.m., and evening workouts got pushed later and later until they were even falling after dinner on some nights. He was training harder than ever but becoming slower.

It just took some outside perspective to recognize the issue: Though his training load had remained the same, the life stress of work (both pressure and hours) and reduced sleep had increased his overall metabolic stress. His body simply couldn't adapt. The solution was tough for him to swallow: I asked him to reduce his overall weekly training load and spend that time sleeping. I also asked him to have a very easy weekend day every other week, replacing that training time with additional sleep, meditation, and recuperation. In other words, I gave him license to be lazy. His weekly training load plummeted from 20 to 22 hours to 13 to 15 hours, but it included specific sessions that included a great deal of high-intensity training.

I was asking him to take a leap of faith. He battled and argued for the first three months of the program, but his complaining slowly dissipated once he began to realize that he was truly enjoying his training again and feeling stronger in workouts. The end result was a return to Kona and a life-best performance relative to his age group.

This is a nice story, but my point is this: How much training is appropriate will be very different at different points in your life, despite the goals being the same. We managed to leverage the fitness this athlete had built over the previous years but reduced his training to keep it effective when his life became busy. The need for such an adjustment is obvious, but many athletes simply don't have the courage to follow the path.

absorb training load. We simply have to acknowledge that, in order to create an effective training plan, we need a dynamic framework that always considers the impact of life stressors on our ability to train hard. I believe that when athletes train by this rule, they make logical decisions about training when managing higher-than-anticipated stress. They typically remain consistent in training, experience less injury, and achieve greater performance gains.

The overall goal is to create a habitual training pattern that includes larger training weeks or blocks when you have more time or capacity, such as a training camp or a holiday. As I've said numerous times, your primary pursuit is *consistency of specific training.* As a working amateur, you have to consider the following important factors when you are deciding on your training load.

Accumulation of life stress. A self-assessment of your current stress and time available for training is the best place to start. These things cannot be easily mapped for you, so your own wisdom and self-awareness are key. Stress and life commitments fluctuate, so reevaluate often.

Individual resilience and training history. Make an honest appraisal of your previous training load, how you cope with training load, and your ability to recover from fatigue. Understand that performance isn't exclusively available to those who train most—you can achieve great results by remaining consistent.

Injury history and risk. Are you a fragile athlete who tends to get injured? Awareness can be the start of mapping a patient program that helps mitigate some of that risk.

Of course, all of these factors require that you set longer-term goals for performance rather than seeking out a fast track to results. My hope is that these guidelines will help you define how and why training fits into your life.

CHARACTERISTICS OF ELITE PERFORMANCE

While amateurs don't have the same goals and training methods as the pros, they can absolutely learn from the characteristics of elite performers in the sport and develop a winning mind-set of their own. Let's move beyond mapping the plan and the logistics of training to investigate the traits of performance.

When you look at any elite performer in the sport, the obvious question is "What makes him or her so special?" Beyond the genetic gifts or talents that provide a platform of opportunity to pursue their dream, the complete answer is more complex. As an elite coach, I am lucky to spend a lot of my time with elite performers and have had the opportunity to learn from them and guide many to success. While every individual is unique, I have identified 10 traits or characteristics that are evident in nearly every one of the more successful elite athletes. There may be more, and many of the traits require development and work in order to become prominent, but they all grow as an athlete develops throughout a career.

1. **Be goal-oriented.** All top athletes have a clear and distinct vision of their path and goals. Goals may evolve over an individual's career, but all athletes achieve positive results by creating and chasing a vision and set of goals.

2. **Commit to ongoing assessment.** Staying on track is key, and the best have great personal reflection and assessment skills but also look outside for guidance and advice. A part of this may include the willingness to review the training approach and to evolve or change it. This takes courage and can occur only for athletes who frequently assess themselves, their setup, and their approach.

3. **Train for specificity.** Keep a laserlike focus on what is important. Great athletes have the ability to carve through the noise of training partners or unsolicited advice and truly focus on executing their plan in pursuit of their goal.

4. **Be resistant to adversity.** One of the key elements I look for in new athletes is their ability to manage and overcome adversity. Triathlon is a demanding sport, and navigation through hard times is the price of admission.

5. **Have patience.** I use the word "journey" to describe the path to elite performance because it doesn't happen instantaneously. Behind every overnight success is many, many years of hard work. This is why patience is a key attribute of every elite performer.

6. **Feed the passion.** You cannot fake this. The high that is brought on by good results doesn't last long, and it won't create the will to embrace the journey and struggle of performance. To excel, you have to fall in love with the process.

7. **Embrace support.** An athlete cannot go it alone. No one person has all the answers, so the best athletes need to be humble enough to build an inner circle of experts to help drive the train forward and maximize their performance. Whether self-coached or supported by many, every elite athlete with lasting success will have mentors, guides, and a support team.

8. **Achieve balance.** The ability to avoid dwelling on success or failure is a magic attribute. Celebrate victories, but keep emotions in check—they should be only as high as the low of struggles or failure of another race or session. This is certainly an area that athletes can learn and improve in, but only if they make the full commitment to do so.

9. **Take calculated risks.** The willingness to take risks can come in many forms but often involves being willing to expose your weaknesses and insecurities and being unafraid of failure. The best athletes are willing to take a risk with purpose in order to reach their desired level.

10. **Make time for recovery.** If you don't establish a platform of health and recovery, you will follow the trajectory of my pro career—plenty of ambition and hard work with a very limited performance yield. I seldom meet an elite athlete who, in time, doesn't appreciate the value of recovery and recuperation as much as hard work and tough intervals. After all, that's the easy part!

I want you to go back and reread the traits above, but this time through a different lens. Think about how these traits relate to different endeavors in your own daily life. We could also identify these traits of elite performance in successful CEOs, concert pianists, the owner of a hugely successful little coffee shop in your town.

I am fortunate to work with leading business executives. I get to know these men and women very well, and they are instrumental in helping me frame my thinking about coaching, guidance, and leadership. Business leaders and professional athletes share similar mind-sets. This isn't surprising because elite performance requires plenty of determination. The gift of physical talent is certainly the ticket to get into the room, but it is these characteristics of performance that help drive the talent toward real and lasting success. Even if you could choose your parents wisely, you would also need to develop these traits to convert potential into performance.

How does this relate to you? Well, you may not be the most genetically gifted swimmer, biker, or runner out there, but that doesn't mean that you can't improve. The long-standing culture of this sport is one of inclusion and self-improvement, and it has never been only about the best. We can determine how we approach the sport (and life). Make it your goal to improve yourself— this is where the magic is, and it is where a winning mind-set is born.

10

Setting Up Your Plan
for Training

As you are now well aware, effective training is not defined simply by work. Any motivated athlete has the ability and potential to work really hard, but the goal should be for that hard work to translate into improved racing and, potentially, life performance. So before we delve into this chapter on a smart way to set up your approach to training, let's remember why we train in the first place. Quite simply, we train in order to gain specific adaptations that prepare us to perform better in our chosen events and races. We want to increase our sustainable pace and power so that we can go faster on the day of the event. This is the framework for our training approach.

I don't want to lead you down a path of belief that less is more (it isn't), but I urge you to remember that more is not always better. We want to do the least amount of training necessary to achieve the desired performance. Now, this concept sounds very simple in hindsight, but the task of planning for effective training is complicated by your background, goals, ability to handle different loads, life situation and stressors, and many other factors. Getting this complex individual recipe right is the Holy Grail of individual training. While no one size will fit all, there are some principles and progressions that can optimize your chances of achieving high-value specific training that progresses toward your goals without compromising performance gains. Just don't buy into the simplistic "more must be better" training approach. The goal is to nail training just right—and the definition of "just right" has to be specific to you, your life, and your goals. Let's explore.

PLANNING THE PHASES OF TRAINING

Many people open a book about training and search for some magical method that will lead to huge breakthrough gains. This might be the chapter that many athletes skip ahead to read: "Tell me what to do, and I will do it!" It is important to realize that, if there is any magic to be had, it will never come in the prescription for workouts or how to set up the season. At purplepatch our framework for seasonal development has been very successful over a wide range of abilities, goals, and time available to train. A good framework will enable you to progress as an athlete while also allowing for individualization and smart decision-making. Do all of my athletes set up their season in the exact progression that I lay out here? Absolutely not. This chapter outlines the most common approach that I deploy and provides you with a great starting point for setting up your season. From there, you need to become an active participant in your own process, be willing to make smart decisions, and tailor the framework to your needs. The magic is in the application of this plan and in the decisions and habits that help support and facilitate it.

In the chapters on swimming, cycling, and running, we explored the phases of training and considered the goals of each phase through the lens of swim-bike-run. What follows is an overview of a typical block of training for each phase. You may recognize key sessions as similar to those in Chapters 6, 7, and 8, here combined with supporting workouts to illustrate the progressive plan.

Post-season (6 to 10 weeks)

Here's the phase that some athletes miss out on altogether, having decided to take a complete break from the sport. Others approach the post-season in a manner that doesn't assist their long-term progression because they eagerly launch back into heavy training, which only sets them up for fatigue or injury early on. I know it's hard to believe that an entire phase of your season should be set aside as preparation to train, but think of the post-season as the platform for your upcoming season, an opportunity to create the readiness to train hard.

There are three main goals to be accomplished in this part of the season:

- Develop technical skills in the three main disciplines
- Improve musculoskeletal resilience to allow heavy training load without injury
- Increase cardiovascular fitness and muscular endurance to a level that facilitates heavy training load

All of these goals are, of course, a part of any phase of training, but I prefer to have athletes view the post-season as preparation to train so that they do not accumulate too much fatigue or try to rush great race-ready fitness. Rather than aiming to be in the highest state of fitness of your life throughout this phase, I want you to aim to do things right. Almost all of your focus should be on holding or improving form and skills and ensuring that all movement patterns are done as well as possible. The last things you should be focusing on are your pace, how much power you can produce, or where you are (in terms of performance) relative to race season. This short phase stresses the opportunity to set skills, technique, and proper habits in place.

Pre-season (10 to 14 weeks)

Here comes the heavy lifting. The pre-season will focus on the progression of fitness and muscular endurance, and the training load is relatively great. Don't mistake this for classic base training, which is typically completed entirely at low intensity with the focus on developing a "base" of aerobic fitness. It's not logical to develop foundational fitness while restricting all other training intensities. I can imagine this approach working for some athletes who respond well to pure endurance training and have unlimited time to train. It simply isn't effective for the vast majority of competing athletes. Besides, athletes work on foundational fitness throughout the season. It is certainly true that fitness takes a long time—measured in years, not months—to develop, but there is no reason to focus purely on low-intensity training at any time of the year.

While the pre-season does focus heavily on low- to medium-intensity training, there is plenty of variance in stress through a variety of cadence and hill work on the bike, strength-related sessions in the swim (such as using buoys and ankle straps, as well as paddles for the more advanced), and hill work in the run. The sessions that might raise eyebrows are those that emphasize very short and high-intensity intervals on both bike and run. These intervals are completed with extended rest, to ensure full recovery, and focus on high recruitment of working muscle and close to max capacity overall effort. A typical session of running might include 6 to 12 repetitions of very high effort, but with a strong focus on posture and technique, lasting 20 to 60 seconds each. Following each high-effort interval would be 3 to 4 minutes at an easy effort to allow complete recovery. The sister session, this time on the bike, would be 6 to 12 repetitions of 1 minute at very high power and cadence, done on a hill or on the flat road. These very-high-intensity efforts are of value only if they are supported with nearly complete recovery between intervals. The gains to be expected from such intervals are:

Muscular recruitment and form. These sessions call for a high recruitment of sport-specific muscle, leaving more fibers available to be utilized in endurance-based sessions. This emphasis correlates with the functional strength work that you will do, which will improve potential muscle to be included in the "usable mix."

Increased endurance capacity. Some research has suggested that these higher-intensity intervals increase the size and number of your mitochondria, which, simply put, are the energy-making factories in your muscle. If this is true, the high-intensity session produces similar results to those hoped for in classic endurance-based sessions.

Improved technique. Assuming that you conduct the very-high-intensity intervals with a supple, fluid approach, the result is improved technical recruitment and pedal stroke.

These sessions are the perfect antidote to the overall endurance focus of the pre-season phase. Assuming that you warm up adequately and execute the intervals correctly, there is no major risk of injury and minimal accumulation of fatigue.

It would be atypical for a week of training to go by without a big-gear, low-cadence, medium-intensity session. Strength-endurance bike sessions are performed on the trainer or on a grade that allows steady and fluid pedaling in a moderately big gear, which means you need to focus on good posture on the bike as well as proper pedal-stroke mechanics. For triathletes, it is preferable for these sessions to be completed in time trial position. Because this is the position used in racing, we are aiming to recruit specific muscles and develop muscular strength and endurance. There are numerous ways to set up intervals with this focus, from a high number of shorter intervals (e.g., 25 × 2 min. Z3 in big gear with 1 min. Z1 fast rpm between intervals) or extended intervals with extended rest (e.g., 4 to 6 × 10 min. Z3 in big gear with 10 min. easy spin between intervals). To begin the phase, I typically maintain the intensity of the intervals, but as the phase progresses and the early races close in, I begin to add strain by progressing intensity either within each interval or by each interval.

A final note on planning: Given the heavy emphasis on endurance, some high-power work, and strength-endurance sessions, it's easy to see that it could be easy for fatigue to accumulate and risk of injury to increase. This is also the time of the season that demands the greatest focus on functional strength training. Don't be surprised if your legs feel heavy during the endurance training. Your twice-weekly strength sessions will entail multiple exercises that call for very high load and short repetitions. Weekly planning and recovery are essential to effective training in the pre-season. This phase becomes very risky if athletes simply dive into the work without adequate conditioning or training. This is where careful preparation starts to pay off. In my experience, conscientious athletes experience moderate risk of injury in this phase, but there is no need to heighten that risk by trying to cram all of the training in without thought of how it should progress or your specific recovery needs. We will address how to go about such planning later in the chapter.

Sustainable Power (4 to 7 weeks)

As the early-season races approach, it's time to transition the focus from building endurance to boosting sustainable speed and power. This is a shorter, transitional phase designed to start from your existing fitness and endurance and begin to sharpen speed and power. The early-season races can be leveraged to support this cause, but the key sessions of each week begin to focus more on a high sustainable effort, often referred to as "above-threshold intervals." At the start of this phase, athletes often report that they feel very fit and strong but not fast. This is no surprise, but this short phase is the catalyst for becoming more race-ready. Though we never lose the focus on form in any session, this phase certainly mostly closely resembles the classic type of interval training. At least one weekly session in each discipline will focus on intervals above maximal steady-state intensity, with little recovery between intervals. Examples would include main sets like these:

- Swim multiple repetitions of 100 to 400 at the strongest effort you can sustain
- Ride 6 to 8 × 4–8 minutes, Zone 4 to Zone 5
- Run 5 to 10 × 1000 meters on the track

This type of work tends to result in very quick boosts of fitness and performance, but it comes at a high cost. Support these sessions with very-low-intensity endurance sessions to provide plenty of recovery. Variance and specificity sharpen as we truly get ready for racing season.

As this phase is completed, I like athletes to take a look back over the previous months of training and preparation. At purplepatch we are fond of saying, "You have built the physiology; now prepare for the race." This is the time for such a cute phrase: All of your training has allowed you to arrive very fit, with more power and improved technical efficiency. Now we enter the race-specific phase, which is the time to prepare for the specific demands of your primary races.

Race-Specific (16 to 24 weeks)

This is perhaps the longest phase of the season. Race-specific preparation signals the greatest divergence in training focus—Ironman athletes pursue a very different training approach than do short-course athletes. The key words remain the same: "familiarity," "pacing development," "dress rehearsal," and "simulators."

By the time you reach this phase of the season, your general foundation of fitness, endurance, and strength should be complete. It is time for training to become highly specific. Of course, this doesn't mean we make each and every session a mini-race simulation, as fatigue would quickly take over and snuff out any potential gains. It is less about working on physiology and more about training to prepare for your ability to race. Fitness can and will still climb, and your performance level will rise, but your range of performance ability will likely narrow toward your key event. Let's compare a sustainable power session to a race-specific session to see what this looks like for an elite athlete.

SUSTAINABLE POWER Swim Main Set	**3 rounds of:** 8 × 100 at best effort with 10 sec. rest 200 easy pull at 60–70% between each set
RACE-SPECIFIC Swim Main Set	**3 to 5 rounds of:** 4 × 50 at 90–95% effort with fast turnover, each with deck-up 400 at 85% with great form 2 × 50 at 90–95%, each with deck-up 100 easy, then 90 sec. rest

The sustainable power set works on improving your sustainable speed, and while it certainly improves your fitness and performance, it doesn't necessarily prepare you for the demands of the event. Let's now consider what happens in the course of a typical swimming race. If you are at all competitive, the start can be a claustrophobic, tumultuous affair. The initial 60 to 120 seconds are performed at a very high intensity, causing your heart rate and breathing to escalate rapidly. It's a battle to maintain strong swimming without exploding. Following the initial burst, the pace tends to settle into a strong, sustainable effort. Your heart rate will continue to be elevated, but the key is not to panic. As the swim portion finishes, you move into position to exit the water and transition from a prone position (swimming) into an upright run.

To do a deck-up, you complete the swim, in this case a 50, then immediately hop out of the pool and stand up. This act elevates the breathing and heart rate, making the next interval highly uncomfortable. The following interval starts from a dive. After two or three of these, you are swimming with a greatly elevated heart and breathing rate, simulating the highly uncomfortable nature of a swim start.

The first three sets of the race-specific sessions are consecutive with no recovery. As you finish one interval, move right into the next. This set truly works on your capacity to control yourself, emotionally and physically, while still maintaining a strong, sustainable effort. This will always be a painful set, but as athletes become familiar with the experience, they tend to panic less. While both the sustainable power and the race-specific main sets include speed and endurance work, the deck-ups simulate the intensity of racing.

PERIODIZATION VERSUS SPECIFIC PROGRESSION

There is always much discussion in coaching and athlete circles about the concept of periodization. A few years ago, "periodization" was the buzzword, though more recently it has lost its appeal. Some coaches casually throw it around to validate their process, while others dismiss it entirely. Periodization originated with Hans Selye's General Adaptation Syndrome, then was popularized through Eastern-bloc training and principles developed by Dr. Tudor Bompa. It was designed to structure a progression of training stimulus to ensure peak performance at or around the time of key events. The idea is fine, but strict application of this model doesn't fit perfectly within the needs of triathlon training.

However, this is not reason enough to dismiss the overall concept out of hand. Let's consider the other extreme: repeating exactly the same type of training week in and week out with limited or no progression of change or stimulus. You would stop gaining positive adaptations relatively quickly—as the body became familiar with the stimulus, the adaptations would be limited. If we simply view periodization as a progression or type of training stimulus that builds over the course of the season, then the concept certainly has legs in the triathlon training approach. I refer to this as specific progression, in contrast to the goal of strict periodization, in which certain phases call for almost the entire focus to be on a specific training stimulus. For example, during an endurance building phase, I don't believe the only goal should be to build endurance. Equally, when there is a focus on sharpening or increasing power, all sessions should not be designed purely around this single goal. The body doesn't respond to such clear-cut specific stimulus, so why try to design your program that way? The lines are murky, and we want to constantly evolve across all areas. This is why I prefer subtle transitions in *emphasis* rather than radical departures in focus and sudden transitions into completely different types of training or load.

So does periodization work? Well, sort of, but it is enough to know that specific progression of training emphasis is essential for you to develop and grow. The question is how to build progression into the phases of your season in a way that allows you to arrive at prime race season more than fit. You want to arrive race-ready!

You should be highly aware of the training stress placed on you by key sessions as well as the supporting sessions that are designed to work on general endurance, help you recover from a previous key session, or allow a bridge effort to set up an upcoming key session. The variance in intensity over the course of weekly training is great, regardless of what race distance you are preparing for. I encourage athletes to clearly identify their weekly key sessions and aim to be ready for their proper execution. To do this, they need to understand how to monitor and manage fatigue and effort in other sessions—this is what being an active participant in your training is all about. There is no more important time of the year to establish and follow great habits of support in sleep, hydration, fueling, nutrition, and recovery than the race-specific phase. This is the phase where you have to be smart, logical, and good at truly following the plan.

SETTING UP YOUR TRAINING BLOCKS

The classic way of setting up training progression is to do three weeks in a row of hard training, or progressively harder training week over week, followed by one week of recovery. This program of training hard, then recovering for an entire week makes it easy for coaches to build training plans and allows athletes to easily identify each week of training as a "build week" or a "recovery week." When it is put into practice, the athlete completes too much training with accumulated fatigue, and other training opportunity is wasted by overrecovery. Not only does this formula absolutely fail to achieve my magic word of training success, "consistency," but also I believe it contributes to a higher risk of injury. In addition, it does not take into account an athlete's resiliency or speed of recovery, let alone how that athlete absorbs workload. Table 10.1 considers a typical scenario by breaking down a cycle of three weeks on, one week off.

TABLE 10.1 | THE CLASSIC APPROACH TO TRAINING

WEEK 1	Initial build
WEEK 2	Build progression
WEEK 3	Big build
WEEK 4	Recovery week

In Week 1, following a prior week of recovery, the athlete is fresh and demolishes training sessions with gusto. An effective training week.

In Week 2, the athlete is still able to absorb and manage the workload; the progressive sessions are challenging, but the training week remains effective. Fatigue accumulates, as by the end of the week the athlete is likely 14 days into an overall build (not all days are high load).

In Week 3, the biggest training-load week is under way, but many of the training sessions are completed with massive fatigue, not with optimal performance. The athlete is hanging on, desperate for the upcoming rest but determined to finish the block. There is little emotional capacity to focus on form, and aches and pains creep in from the accumulation of fatigue. Training becomes ineffective.

In Week 4, the athlete is so physically and emotionally spent that they fall into the recovery week with delight, often wanting to escape the torture of that last daunting week. The athlete bounces back and feels fresh after three to four days but keeps recovering for the full week to ensure readiness for the next three-week cycle. An entire week of desperate recovery results in ineffective training.

And so the cycle continues, with about half of the total training opportunity providing effective training. The other half is marked by the great peaks and valleys of fatigue that limit triathlon performance. Our mission is to find rhythm and consistency. While you should accumulate fatigue, and you will endure days (or even blocks of days) of feeling tired, the highs and lows created by this approach are what we want to avoid.

There are multiple routes to performance, but I suggest that you abandon this outdated approach and get in front of the fatigue with regular short breaks for recuperation and recovery. These minibreaks can be one to four days of recuperation—just enough to prevent the accumulation of too much fatigue, which leaves the athlete desperate for recovery and devalues training for several days in a row. Because our mind-set is all about achieving long-term consistency and accumulating as much effective training as possible over an extended period, properly integrated minirecovery is critical.

Of course each athlete will respond to training, as well as recovery, in a different manner. Certain trends and generalizations do occur that apply to most athletes, and we use these to build the main framework, but we cannot declare any one method to be the Holy Grail. There must be some flexibility and ongoing assessment in the execution. Table 10.2 shows a training block

TABLE 10.2 | **THE TYPICAL ATHLETE'S TRAINING BLOCK**

DAY 1	**Build** (intervals)
DAY 2	**Build** (endurance)
DAY 3	**Build** (intervals)
DAY 4	**Light/recovery**
DAY 5	**Build** (intervals)
DAY 6	**Build** (endurance/intervals)
DAY 7	**Light/recovery**
DAY 8	**Build** (intervals)
DAY 9	**Build** (endurance)
DAY 10	**Build** (intervals)
DAY 11	**Light/recovery**
DAY 12	**Light/recovery**
DAY 13	**Build** (endurance)
DAY 14	**Light/recovery**

Note: On Day 13 we can sneak in a higher-load session that can be extended throughout the season. During the race-specific phase, a race or race simulation works well on this day.

for an athlete who responds in a typical manner. Instead of delving into the specifics of the days and sessions, this two-week snapshot simply highlights the big picture of progressive training. After completing the block, the athlete would go on and repeat the pattern for one or two more cycles of training.

This progression isn't universal—some athletes are more fragile, whereas others are highly resilient. I have coached both types, and of the two examples that come to mind, both are highly successful Ironman champions. One tends to be extremely resilient, responding to rest very quickly, while the other has less musculoskeletal resilience and requires plenty of recovery between blocks of work. Let's explore how their training progressions differ from the norm in Tables 10.3 and 10.4.

TABLE 10.3 | **THE RESILIENT ATHLETE'S TRAINING BLOCK**

DAY 1	**Build** (intervals)
DAY 2	**Build** (endurance)
DAY 3	**Build** (intervals)
DAY 4	**Light/recovery**
DAY 5	**Build** (intervals)
DAY 6	**Build** (endurance/intervals)
DAY 7	**Build** (intervals)
DAY 8	**Light/recovery**
DAY 9	**Build** (intervals)
DAY 10	**Build** (endurance)
DAY 11	**Build** (intervals)
DAY 12	**Light/recovery**
DAY 13	**Light/recovery**
DAY 14	**Build** (endurance)

Note: *The final endurance session completes the cycle, and we bridge to three more days of progression.*

Light/Recovery Days

Days designated as light/recovery are not wasted training days, and they should not be spent simply lying on the couch. In fact, if energy allows, many athletes will continue with relatively strong swimming sessions on these days. Furthermore, there is high value to be derived from the lighter endurance, skills development, and light speed work that may fill these sessions. They can vary from very little training to simply less-stressful training, but each session has a place in bridging consistency.

The real flexibility enters when bridging from one cycle to the next—this is where you have to be an active participant in your own process and make smart decisions about your readiness to return to full load. If you typically

TABLE 10.4 | **THE FRAGILE ATHLETE'S TRAINING BLOCK**

DAY 1	**Build** (intervals)
DAY 2	**Build** (endurance)
DAY 3	**Light/recovery** (intervals)
DAY 4	**Build** (intervals)
DAY 5	**Build** (endurance)
DAY 6	**Light/recovery**
DAY 7	**Build** (intervals)
DAY 8	**Build** (endurance)
DAY 9	**Light/recovery**
DAY 10	**Build** (endurance)
DAY 11	**Build** (intervals)
DAY 12	**Light/recovery**
DAY 13	**Light/recovery** (optional endurance day)
DAY 14	**Light/recovery**

Note: Depending on how things are going, Day 13 may become an optional endurance build day. In the final three days of lighter work, swim load can be maintained, but running stress should be limited. We may retain frequency of running but drop any intervals.

require one day or more of lighter training before returning to full load, that will nearly always be a smart decision, as it prevents low-quality training and reduces your risk of sickness and injury.

The Value of Repeating Sessions

Within the cycle of training you adopt, there will be multiple key sessions. When you repeat the cycle, then repeat it (potentially) a third time, the sessions can be very similar. These sessions will include a main set that is the same as the one completed a week or two earlier but will evolve the load through extended duration, number of intervals, or other variables. In rare instances, such as when the initial session was very challenging, I may prescribe exactly the same main set for my athletes. This is not lazy coaching, as there is nothing better for adaptation than repeating the stress, albeit with a slightly higher load. It also provides you with an opportunity to redo a session that has already been completed. The initial run-through of a brand-new session may not always yield optimal training performance—some emotional resources are allocated to navigating an unfamiliar program. By the second time, the progression is more familiar, and you bring to it the wisdom of your initial session. Your mind and body understand the stress and are well suited for optimal execution. My athletes are used to my prescribing a main set they have already completed. The goal and instructions are always to aim to repeat it with perfection.

DEFINING YOUR WORKOUTS

You can foster a more nimble decision-making process relative to the framework if you understand the key sessions within each week. Training consistency is critical, and all training has its place, but within each week there is a weighted emphasis on sessions that are central to the focus of that phase and that particular week. The other sessions are still important, but they act as the supporting cast. Defining these and understanding the purpose create clarity for you as an athlete. It is obvious that the time to be "on" is during the foundational sessions. If life strikes a blow, we aim to hold on to these sessions as much as possible within the context of the block of work. The supporting sessions are made up of general endurance, skills, and bridge sessions, so if a workout needs to be skipped, it should be a supporting session that gets the chop.

Defining the sessions also helps athletes to follow the plan as intended. Most supporting sessions will not include massive physical stress, so they offer an opportunity to focus on form, minimize stress, and allow recovery. Knowing this, a dedicated athlete is less likely to go crazy with intensity in these sessions. Learning when to be "on" and when to be "off" is good practice that extends into race performance.

Key Sessions

By defining a workout's goal or purpose, athletes are more likely to follow the prescription and purpose of the session rather than drift into work that is too easy or too challenging. I like to build training around key sessions that act as the bedrock of the week. Depending on the particular phase of training, the load of these sessions can vary greatly, but you will always know that these are the sessions with great specificity and purpose, the ones to be ready for, and the ones you should try not to miss. This doesn't mean that they will always leave you with a reservoir of fatigue. In fact, in the post-season, this session may be purely skills development and light endurance, challenging you emotionally but not inviting fatigue.

A simple rule of thumb is that there are typically six key sessions within each week of training—that is, two sessions for each discipline: swim, bike, and run. The length of each session is not important, but the fact that there are at least six sessions is! Lining up these sessions across the phases of training can be a nice way to view the progression. In the sport-specific chapters (Chapters 6, 7, and 8), we considered examples of key sessions within each phase of the progression. In the sample training blocks at the end of this chapter, the key sessions are highlighted.

Supporting Sessions

Because your supporting sessions bookend the key sessions of the week, allow recovery, bridge to an upcoming session, or work in high-value general endurance and skills development that create less fatigue, they are integral to the fabric of the program. I often think of supporting sessions as the unsung heroes of the training plan, as they can promote consistency, prevent injury, and minimize the accumulation of fatigue. Naturally, this means you must embrace the concept of lighter sessions rather than giving in to the temptation to add duration or intensity. At purplepatch we have a mantra to reinforce this point: "It takes courage to recover." No truer statement can be made about training. I have little problem compelling a highly motivated athlete to get out there and train hard. Most athletes don't need to be persuaded of the merits of tough sessions; the "stick" doesn't come out very often. Instead, it's my job to rein in athletes from their desire to excel and improve.

This reality is rooted in the fact that lighter sessions or days don't deliver the same validation, buzz, or confidence. Following a tough foundational session, we feel great, as if we truly accomplished something. The supporting session falls well short of this high. It takes an athlete with true vision and confidence to realize that these lighter sessions and days are a part of a greater plan. It is not laziness; it is not a shortcut—it is truly part of the essential fabric of training progression.

In Appendix C you'll find different templates for how to structure key sessions and supporting sessions within a week of training. You can select a template that fits with your lifestyle and schedule and then build out your training from there.

COMING BACK FROM REST

Throughout the training process, you will need to back off and recuperate. Whether it is one or two easy sessions or complete rest days, this healing is critical to facilitate adaptations, allow healing, and emotionally rejuvenate. The aspect that is seldom discussed is how you will typically feel *following* this rest.

When you take rest, or have a few light days, it is not uncommon to feel truly awful. You may feel lethargic, flat, and completely unfit. This feeling can be disconcerting and may even affect your confidence, and it is one of the reasons many highly motivated athletes struggle to embrace rest and recovery. You build in the recovery in hopes of better performance only to head out on a run and feel like a donkey dipped in cement. Don't worry; this is a result of the hormonal response from rest, and it is a part of the healing process. If you wait long enough, your next session might feel sprightly and sharp, but that would not be the smartest way to achieve performance. Instead, you need to take some steps to offset this feeling and reestablish your training rhythm as quickly as possible.

Warm-up. Double the length of your warm-up in the first session back—this is the single best thing you can do. Progressively build the effort over the warm-up to allow your body to respond. A longer warm-up is especially important if you have intervals.

Start with endurance. If possible, focus the first session on endurance. If you need to do intervals, begin with progressive building intervals.

Accept and anticipate. You might get lucky and have no feeling of lethargy, but knowledge is power. If your body feels awful after rest, remember that this indicates healing and thus adaptations. Don't run away from it—embrace it.

DEALING WITH TRAVEL

One of the big hurdles of a triathlete's life is dealing with travel, for racing or work, while also finding time to train. Here are some tips that might help ease the burden and negative effects of travel.

Hydration and nutrition. There is little doubt that proper hydration before, during, and after travel can help prevent the negative effects that occur. We see better results when athletes eat foods that are higher in protein for both an inflight snack and the meal following a flight. Much of this benefit may be attributed to the fact that protein can reduce cortisol, your stress hormone.

Compression and movement. Flying is a good time to wear compression socks. Whether they are truly effective or simply a placebo, most athletes report a positive effect from flying in compression. Just don't wear full-lower-body compression tights all the way through a flight to Brazil with two layovers, as I once did. I ended up sweaty and uncomfortable, and the effect was certainly not worth any possible positive results! As annoying as it might be to your neighbors, moving frequently around the cabin is a massive advantage. Sitting is one of the most corrosive things we do, so get up and move around as much as you can.

On arrival, get moving. Low-intensity exercise, whether walking, running, swimming, or riding, helps move blood and facilitate recovery.

Allow one day per time zone. If you are crossing time zones for a race, a simple and effective rule of thumb is to travel one day in advance of the event for every time zone you will cross. Admittedly, this is not always possible, but it is a good guideline.

Give yourself time to recover. Even if you are simply traveling for work, you must respect the effects of travel. To maintain overall consistency, I tell athletes to embrace at least one day of endurance-focused work before diving back into tough interval-based training.

ADAPTING YOUR PLAN

This all looks great on paper, but the one thing this framework doesn't consider is the radically changing dynamics of real life as well as your actual response to training stress. What happens if you get sick? Should you take a lighter day even if you are feeling great? What about integrating travel for racing? Quite simply, it is impossible for you to force yourself into such a rigid framework without the tools to navigate through real-life commitments, fatigue, or other factors that intervene. I always encourage athletes to simply use these suggestions as a general guide to steer them through the progression. The best athletes will be active participants who will adapt the plan based on their own individual situations or fatigue level. Of course this is no easy task; it takes wisdom and courage to make logical decisions on whether to push on or pull back.

What if I Get Sick During Training?

This is an area where logic must always trump emotion. I encourage athletes to retreat from the myopic lens of the next workout and take a longer-term view of what we are trying to accomplish. Remember that training is a physiological stress, albeit an essential one designed to create adaptations. If you are sick, you are under 24/7 physiological stress that is more than likely going to greatly hinder or prevent positive physiological adaptations to that training stress. For this reason, I seldom ask athletes to train at their usual level through sickness. This doesn't mean you should jump into bed at the first sign of a sniffle. Our whole mission is to limit the time you are burdened by sickness, and the best antidote tends to be as much rest and sleep as possible, as well as plenty of fluids and high-quality nutrition. After that, it becomes all about patience. If you have symptoms that are systemic in nature, or you feel the sickness in your body (fever, chills), or you have a chest infection, then complete rest is necessary. If you have symptoms that include only a runny nose, sniffles, or a slight sore throat, you can likely maintain exercise, but avoid all intervals or high intensity. You also want to keep the duration of training relatively short. My rule of thumb is nothing over Zone 2 and nothing over 45 minutes.

What if I Have Been Sick?

After you recover from sickness, how do you adapt the plan and get yourself back into training? The worst thing you can do is dive immediately back into tough intervals on the first day that you feel better. Taking it slowly requires plenty of patience, but I ask athletes to wait two or three days before ramping back up into training.

DAY 1	Light activity and low intensity. A small ride and run without intensity of real effort. Monitor how you feel and respond afterward.
DAY 2	A full day of training, but all endurance-focused with no intervals. If all goes well, hop right back into a regular training schedule.
DAY 3	If you had any doubts after day 2, take one more endurance day then return to your plan on day 4.

When illness occurs, you will want to look back and see what key sessions you missed in your training when you were struck down. You then have to decide how to shift the plan around to fit in these sessions or whether it is better to simply move on.

Just remember that there is not an Olympic or world champion who hasn't gone through their training and racing life without plenty of bouts of sickness—it is a part of the journey. Remaining logical and taking a broader view of your training will help you navigate through without desperation.

What if I Get Injured Running?

Let's face it, the vast majority of overuse injuries occur in running, and it is an issue of continuing frustration for many athletes. There are a few points to keep in mind regarding injuries that are often the result of running.

Is it from the bike? Always check your riding cleats to see if they have shifted or moved, or think back to consider whether you have evolved your riding position, cleats, pedals, or anything else that may influence your musculoskeletal integrity.

Is the injury merely a symptom? More often than not, the location where you feel the pain is not where the issue is actually originating. Getting to the source of the problem is key to rehab, recovery, and future injury prevention. For example, a tight IT band is often the symptom of a problem that originates in the lower back or hips. Look up or down from the problem to find a solution. A good professional therapist can assist you.

The foam roller is "prehab," not rehab! While foam rollers, TriggerPoint massage balls, and other methods are great for maintenance, they are not designed to replace a professional therapist. If you have a niggling ache or pain, don't dive onto that spot and attack it vigorously. Your foam roller can't cure your injury. Simply maintain an overall-body approach (see "Self-Massage Protocol for Recovery," page 59) that targets all areas, and either rest or seek help. As discussed, the pain is not always at the location of the cause, so don't attack it.

The good news is that it is triathlon. This is not a single-session sport, so even if you are sidelined with an injury in running, you still have massive opportunities to grow and evolve. I prefer athletes to focus on what they *can* do instead of what they cannot. If one sport requires rest, focus on the other two and evolve them.

Do what you can do. If running is out of the question, there are often other activities that can *help your running*. Riding provides good cross-pollination for running performance, but aqua-jogging and the elliptical trainer can be good substitutions. You may even be lucky enough to have access to more modern alternatives, such as underwater and AlterG treadmills, but utilize them under the guidance of a professional.

Do aqua-jogging right. Your aqua-jogging sessions will *feel* easier, and it will be tough to get your heart rate up as high as during regular running. This is due to the non-weight-bearing nature of the activity and the hydrostatic pressure of water. Make most sessions relatively short and focused on higher-intensity intervals. There is little point in doing long, slow distance during aqua-jogging.

Returning to running. When you are ready to evolve back into running, plan a *more than patient* progression that includes shorter sessions with walk breaks. Depending on the injury, I often deploy a 45-day protocol designed to bring the athlete back into complete run training. Forty-five days! Yes, taking that amount of time requires patience, but if you follow this protocol, you will have a much better chance of getting back to running without another flare-up of the same injury.

TROUBLESHOOTING TRAINING & PERFORMANCE

If your training is not translating to improvements, don't automatically blame yourself, your coach, or the training. First, determine whether there are *life factors* that are getting in the way of training adaptations. Take an honest look at your life to assess whether there has been an increase in stress, disruption of sleep patterns, or a change in your approach to eating . . . or anything else that could be causing changes to your approach or an increase in stress.

Determine whether you are overstressed or fatigued. Are you simply tired? Keep an eye out for all the cues and symptoms that show that you are overtired and unable to perform. Do you experience night sweats or sleepless nights, retention of body fat, loss of motivation, fatigue during the day (at work), or unusually sore muscles? If so, you are likely underrecovering or training too hard given your current life situation.

Evaluate your plan and application. I find that when it comes to training sessions, many athletes try to throw the kitchen sink into every single week. As we are accustomed to our seven-day cycle, most athletes aim to fit *every type of training into every single week*—a long ride, long run, bike intervals, hill reps on the run, the big swim, and much more. This approach often leads to an overload of training stress because there is not adequate time to recuperate from a key session and prepare for the next. It is not that the sessions themselves are bad; there are simply too many of them in a compressed time.

Are you overmeasuring and underfeeling? With the introduction of so many quantitative devices (GPS, heart rate monitors, and power meters), many athletes have forgotten how to *feel* their effort and training. Measuring is easy, but learning how to truly feel in training is incredibly hard. The backlash against measuring tools is in full effect as many overfocus on and are guided by these tools without listening to the signals the body provides. I encourage athletes to utilize these tools as governors and feedback tools but hesitate to have them employ the tools to determine effort. The engineers and measuring fanatics will kick and scream, but performance is not a simplistic calculation. Disregard your internal clock and perceived effort, and you will never truly evolve as an athlete.

Step away. If you are struggling, and not getting the results you expect, you may simply need a break. It doesn't mean you have to stop training or chasing your goals, but a week or two of less structure, or training simply by feel, can help you reset your mind and body. If you do take a step away, be open to evolving your approach. I am always amazed at how rigid many coaches and athletes can be about their approach to training.

What if I Lose My Performance in Power or Speed Workouts?

If you feel "flat" when performing lots of higher-intensity or speed workouts, the solution is likely not what you may think. Back in my swimming days, we used to say, "If the sprinters are not sprinting well, train them with the distance crew." It wasn't that simple, as real distance-based training would have depleted the sprinters, but the point was this: To find speed, first take it away.

If you are consistently underperforming in your speed or high-intensity work, do multiple days in a row of lower-intensity endurance training. Maintain just a little neuromuscular work, with strides or spin-ups, but keep the stress and speed minimal. The likelihood is that within a week or two, the speed will come right back to you.

What if My Swimming Performance Isn't Improving?

Commit to it. I generally like athletes to focus on improving their strengths, but the swim is a worthy project for any serious triathlete. This is a tough concept to grasp, as the swim takes up the least time in the race and the available time gains may be limited, but the positives are too strong to ignore. If your swim is a true weakness, then I suggest mapping a two- to three-year commitment, especially in the winter months, and aiming to turn yourself into a swimmer. Here are a few pointers on how to successfully go about it:

Don't go it alone. Swim in a competitive group environment that is focused on triathlon. It's unlikely that you will achieve the desired improvements on your own.

Don't fixate on technique. Don't try to turn yourself into a pure swimmer, and don't focus only on drills and stroke work. Muscular endurance and real swimming are key. Figure out the fundamentals of technique, then work hard. It is more simple than you think.

Use your swim toys. The snorkel, buoy, and ankle strap are tools that help force proper technique *while you are training;* hence, you kill two birds with one stone. Drills should be minimal.

Use swimming as rehab. Too many athletes struggle to truly take the required rest to allow recovery following the beating the body takes in the season. Focusing on swimming while reducing run training typically allows musculoskeletal recovery and reduces your risk of injury in the next season. There are fewer injuries in swimming, and the leg muscles have plenty of time to heal.

Commit to becoming a better athlete. I have yet to see any athlete fail to improve as a triathlete as a result of embracing a swim project. You'll take invaluable lessons from the experience—your internal clock, pacing, patience, and overall conditioning. Every one of my athletes who has truly committed to swimming has improved globally as a triathlete. Don't run away from it! This swimming project helped Jesse Thomas fast-track emotionally as a triathlete while also preventing him from focusing too much on his established strength (running). It helped him understand training and become a great triathlete.

What if I Am Training Hard but Cannot Lose Body Fat?

Whenever this occurs, the inclination is for the athlete to go on some form of intervention or diet, but this approach is seldom the solution. Before you evolve your eating habits, you should first review your training load relative to life stress (as discussed throughout this book!) and ensure that you are fueling adequately following each workout and eating *enough* calories to support your training. Once you have gone through this process, you can begin to consider interventions. If you aim to improve body composition, success can come from front-loading your calories (consuming more early in the day and never getting into early deficits), then reducing your starchy carbohydrate allowance later in the day. If there is a time and place for deficits, it is during your evening meal, when you focus only on vegetables, a high-quality protein source, and some high-quality fat. If you support your training with postexercise fueling, get enough calories throughout the day, and restrict starchy carbohydrates and sugar in the evening, you will likely evolve. One final thought: Commit to the long term, and commit to habits. I am not a fan of trying to hit "race weight." The scales don't drive the decisions; good habits, high-quality fueling and eating, and smart training do.

SAMPLE TRAINING BLOCKS

I have outlined a two-week training block for each phase of training. You will notice that there is a similar template from one week to the next. Some workouts remain relatively similar, while others evolve in focus. The key sessions will look similar to the sample workouts provided in the sport-specific chapters.

As you plan your own progressive program, please keep in mind that the purpose of these sample training blocks is to provide examples of focus and training progression. What follows is not a personal training plan that will be suitable for every reader. Other considerations:

- All of these training blocks are a snapshot of two weeks over the course of a progressive program. In a complete plan, there would be progressive training blocks building to each of these two-week periods and/or progressing thereafter.
- Most sessions provide detail only for the main set. Remember to include a proper warm-up and skills development or preparatory pre–main set where appropriate.
- The template was created to suit a range of athletes; however, the training load would be too high (in number of sessions) for a very busy professional and too low (in sessions and duration) for an elite athlete. You may need to scale up or down.
- The template does not consider individual needs or points of emphasis (for example, sport-specific weaknesses).
- Cycling sessions need to be adapted if you rely on trainer-based sessions in the winter months because of limited time or inclement weather.

Treat your plan for training as a "live" document—ongoing assessment of fatigue, history, and focus is critical, and sessions should be adjusted as needed.

Key workouts are highlighted; these are the sessions you don't want to miss. Refer to Appendix C (page 335) for more options on how to structure key workouts within the training week.

	KEY SWIM
	KEY RIDE
	KEY RUN

SAMPLE TRAINING BLOCK FOR POST-SEASON

	WORKOUT 1	WORKOUT 2
M	**Optional SWIM** Focus on technique, some light 25s at speed (high rest), and nothing stressful.	**Optional RIDE** 45–120 min. light, easy ride with higher rpm, smaller gear.
T	**Key SWIM** 20 to 40 × 100. Alternate 5 sets with snorkel, buoy, band at 70%; 5 sets swim at 80% transferring good form; repeat until done. All with 10 sec. rest between intervals.	**Functional Strength +** **Key RUN Endurance** 30–75 min. Z2 with walk breaks as needed. Every 5th minute surge to Z4 with cues for great form.
W	**RIDE Endurance** 90–120 min. Initial 30 min. fast rpm in small gear. *Focus on posture and pedal stroke.* **RUN Off the Bike** 15–25 min. low stress (musculoskeletal load).	**P.M. OFF**
T	**Key SWIM** 3 to 6 rounds of 200 snorkel, buoy, ankle strap at 70%; 2 × 100 snorkel and ankle strap at 80%; 4 × 50 swim great form at 80–85%. Rest 10 sec. throughout sets, no break between rounds. **+ Functional Strength**	**Key RIDE Strength** 3 to 5 × 10 min. at Z3 on 3–5% grade all big gear, 40–60 rpm. Stand at least 3–4 times on each grade to regain momentum with up to 10 pedal strokes. 5 min. spin-down between intervals.
F	**RUN** 30–50 min. Low stress with no intervals. Walk breaks are still OK.	**P.M. OFF**
S	**SWIM** 8 to 12 × 100–150 snorkel, buoy, band at 70%; 8 to 12 × 75–125 snorkel and band at 75–80%; 8 to 12 × 50–100 swim great form at 80–85%. Rest 15 sec. throughout sets, 1 min. between rounds.	**Key RUN** 30–50 min. Z1/2 to Z2, then 6 × 30–40 sec. blast Z4/5 to Z5 on 4–6% grade with great form. Walk downhill for 2 min. rest between efforts. *Focus on high-stress power intervals with great form. Complete rest between intervals is essential.*
S	**Key RIDE Endurance** Up to 4.5 hr. Low stress as long as you wish. *Reduction of physical stress leaves capacity for emotional focus on skills, gears, pedaling.* **RUN Off the Bike** 3 × 9 min. Z2, with 1 min. walk to recover (musculoskeletal load).	**P.M. OFF**

	WORKOUT 1	WORKOUT 2
M	**Optional SWIM** 3 to 5 rounds of 200–400 snorkel, buoy, ankle strap at 70%; 8 × 25 odds easy, evens fast with good form. *Focus on form and light speed.*	**Optional RIDE Light** 45–90 min. all at higher rpm, small gear. *Focus on recovery and skills.* Finish with cornering skills in parking lot.
T	**Key SWIM** 3 to 5 rounds of 8 to 12 × 25 ankle strap and snorkel at 80% with 10 sec. rest, right into 200–400 swim (snorkel optional) at 70% endurance with 1 min. rest. *Focus on creating taut body and alignment.*	**Functional Strength +** **Key RUN** 6 to 10 × 10-sec. strides following warm-up. 40–60 min. Z1/2, walk 30 sec. every 6th min. *Focus on form.*
W	**RIDE Endurance** 1.5–2 hr. Initial 30 min. fast rpm, small gear. *Focus on posture and pedal stroke.*	**Optional RUN** 15–40 min. Z1/2 to Z2, low stress for musculoskeletal resilience.
T	**Key SWIM** 20 to 40 × 50 (¼ snorkel and ankle strap, ¼ snorkel, ¼ snorkel and ankle strap, ¼ swim): all at 70 to 80%, with 5–7 sec. rest between intervals. *Focus on alignment, stroke rate, and good form while building endurance.*	**Key RIDE Strength** 10 to 20 × 2 min. Z3 at 35–50 rpm on shallow grade (3–5%), spin 1 min. between each interval. *Focus on pedal stroke, posture, transitions in/out of the saddle for form and skills.*
F	**REST DAY** **Optional RUN** 10–30 min. shake-out run for the soul. *No real focus here.*	**P.M. OFF**
S	**RUN** 40–60 min. low stress, all Z1/2 with the last 2 min. of each 5 min. focused on posture, foot speed, and body position. *Use Tempo Trainer to keep foot speed at lighter effort.*	**P.M. OFF**
S	**Key SWIM** 3 to 5 rounds of 8 to 12 × 25 ankle strap and snorkel at 80% with 10 sec. rest; 200–400 swim endurance (snorkel optional) at 70% with 1 min. rest. *Focus on creating taut body and alignment.*	**Key RIDE Endurance** Up to 3 hr. Z2 with Z2/3 on hills, not deep, preferably on road bike. *Focus on form, standing transitions, cornering.* **RUN Off the Bike** 5–30 min. for musculoskeletal resilience.

SAMPLE TRAINING BLOCK FOR PRE-SEASON

	WORKOUT 1	WORKOUT 2
M	**Optional SWIM** Light 25s at speed (high rest), nothing stressful. *Focus on technique.* 2 to 5 rounds of 300 snorkel at 70%; 4 × 50 progress sets 1–4 to fast; 2 × 25 sprint fast.	**RUN** Up to 1 hr. low stress with nothing over Z2. Walk breaks as needed.
T	**Key SWIM** 10 × 100 snorkel, buoy, ankle strap at 70% with 10 sec. rest; 20 × 50 snorkel at 80% (paddles for advanced swimmers) with 10 sec. rest; 40 × 25 at 90% swim with great form and stroke rate (Tempo Trainer) with 5 sec. rest.	**Key RUN** 10 × 1 min. Z5 on 5–9% grade. Rest 3 min. to completely recover between efforts. *Focus on proper form throughout.*
W	**RIDE Endurance** 90 min.–3 hr. Initial 30 min. fast rpm, small gear. *All focus on posture and pedal stroke.* **RUN Off the Bike** 15–25 min. low stress (musculoskeletal load).	P.M. OFF
T	**Key SWIM** 3 to 6 rounds of 6 × 100 snorkel, buoy, ankle strap at 75% with 10 sec. rest; right into 400 swim at 85% (paddles for advanced swimmers) with 30 sec. rest. **+ Functional Strength**	**Key RIDE Endurance** 75–120 min. on trainer. Warm up, then ride 60 min. continuous as 6 rounds of 2 min. Z2 choice rpm; 2 min. Z2/3 dropping rpm; 3 min. Z2/3 at 50 rpm; 2 min. Z2/3 ramping rpm; 1 min. Z1 fast rpm. *Focus on variance of rpm and mechanical fatigue.*
F	**RUN Low Intensity** 30–70 min. low stress with no intervals. Walk breaks are still OK.	P.M. OFF
S	**SWIM** 24 × 75–200, 4 sets with snorkel, buoy, ankle strap at 70%; 4 sets swim at 80%; 4 sets with snorkel, buoy, ankle strap at 70%; 4 sets swim at 85%; 4 sets with snorkel, buoy, ankle strap at 70%; 4 sets swim with paddles at 90%. All with 10–15 sec. rest between intervals.	**Key RUN Hilly Endurance** 50–90 min. Z3+ on hills with good form. **OR Tempo Maintenance RUN** 15–20 × 2 min. at Z2 with 1 min. easy Z1/2 walk between intervals. *Pace is not high, just form-based muscle recruitment.*
S	**Key RIDE Strength** 90 min.–4 hr. After warm-up, ride 3 to 6 × 10 min. Z3 bigger gear TT position, 35–55 rpm, into 10 min. spin Z1 light. **+ Functional Strength**	P.M. OFF

	WORKOUT 1	WORKOUT 2
M	**Optional SWIM** 3 to 5 rounds of 200–400 snorkel, buoy, ankle strap at 70%; right into 8 × 25, odds easy, evens fast with good form. *Focus on form and light speed.*	**Optional RIDE Light** 1–2 hr. All higher rpm and small gear for recovery and skills only. Finish with cornering skills in parking lot.
T	**Key SWIM** 4 × 600–1000, set 1 as snorkel, buoy, ankle strap at 70%; set 2 as 2 × 300–500 at 75% with snorkel; set 3 as 4 × 150–250 at 80%; set 4 as 10 × 100 short rest at 85% with paddles (Tempo Trainer for stroke rate).	**Key RIDE** 6 to 10 × 1 min. Z4/5 fast with 4 min. spin between intervals.
W	**RUN Endurance** Up to 90 min. smooth and controlled Z2 run. Walk breaks as needed. **+ Functional Strength**	**Optional RIDE** 60–120 min. low stress for foundational endurance.
T	**Key SWIM** 2 to 4 rounds of 300–600 smooth, swim every 3rd 100 with fast stroke rate; right into 12 to 16 × 25. *Different focus on FAST swimming each round:* **round 1** as odds fast, evens easy; **round 2** as 2 fast, 1 easy; **round 3** as 3 fast, 1 easy; **round 4** with fins, all fast with lots of rest.	**Key RIDE Strength** 10 to 20 × 2 min. Z3 at 35–50 rpm on shallow grade (3–5%) with 1 min. easy spin between each interval. *Focus on form and skills: pedal stroke, posture, some transitions in/out of saddle.*
F	**REST DAY** **Optional RUN** 30–50 min. shake-out run for the soul. *No real focus here.*	**Optional SWIM** Very low stress, all form-based.
S	**RUN** 50–80 min. all Z1/2 with the last 2 min. of each 5 min. focused on posture, foot speed, and body position. *Use Tempo Trainer to keep foot speed at lighter effort.* **+ Functional Strength**	**P.M. OFF**
S	**Key SWIM Endurance** 3 to 6 rounds of 200 at 70%; 2 × 150 at 80%; 3 × 100 at 85%. Rest 5–7 sec. for all sets, no break between rounds. *Mix in pulling gear as needed.*	**Key RIDE Endurance** Up to 5 hr. Z2 with Z2/3 on hills, not deep, preferably on road bike. *Focus on form, standing transitions, cornering.* **RUN Off the Bike** 15–40 min. light for musculoskeletal resilience.

SAMPLE TRAINING BLOCK FOR SUSTAINABLE POWER

	WORKOUT 1	WORKOUT 2
M	**RUN Low Stress** Up to 60 min. with nothing over Z2. Walk breaks as needed.	**RIDE Low Stress** Up to 2 hr. all Z1/2 easy effort.
T	**Key SWIM** 4 × 600–1000, set 1 as pull with snorkel, buoy, ankle strap; set 2 as 6 to 10 × 100 at 80% on short rest; set 3 as 2 × 300–500 pull at 70%; set 3 as 6 to 10 × 100 best effort with 45 sec. rest.	**Key RUN** 6 to 10 × 4 min. at best sustained effort across all intervals with 4 min. rest between each interval. *This is a very challenging session—hold form under duress.*
W	**RIDE Endurance** 90 min.–3 hr. Initial 30 min. fast rpm, small gear. All focused on posture and pedal stroke. *(Note the effort needs to drop here, as the key sessions are such high load.)* **RUN Off the Bike** 15–25 min., low stress (musculoskeletal load).	**P.M. OFF**
T	**Key SWIM** 2 to 4 × super 500 broken swims (25, 50, 75, 100, 100, 75, 50, 25). All fast with 15 sec. rest between intervals. Between 500s swim 6 × 50 easy with buoy to recover. Finish with 500 for time. **+ Functional Strength**	**Key RIDE Muscle Tension** (on trainer) 2 to 5 × 4 min., 2 to 5 × 3 min., 2 to 5 × 2 min., 2 to 5 × 1 min. All Z2/3 to Z3 at 35–55 rpm with 1 min. Z1 fast rpm between intervals. Then 1 × 10–30 min. Z2 endurance focus with good pedaling.
F	**RUN Low Intensity** 30–70 min. low stress with no intervals. Walk breaks are still OK.	**P.M. OFF**
S	**SWIM** 12 × 200–400 progress by sets of 3, with the last 3 at best effort. All with only 30 sec. rest between intervals. *Note this is a threshold session.*	**Key RIDE Power** 90 min.–4 hr. Warm up, then ride 3 × 6 min. progress effort 1 to 3 to best effort; 3 × 5 min. at the last 6 min. power, 3 × 4 min. at the last 5 min. power, 3 × 3 min. at the last 4 min. power. All with rest equal to interval.
S	**Key RUN Endurance** 50–75 min. Z1/2 to Z2, low stress. *Nothing deep at all.* **+ Functional Strength**	**P.M. OFF**

	WORKOUT 1	WORKOUT 2
M	**Optional SWIM** 3 to 5 rounds of 200–400 snorkel, buoy, ankle strap at 70%; right into 8 × 25 with odds easy, evens fast with good form. *All focused on form and light speed.*	**Optional RIDE Light** 1–2 hr. all higher rpm and small gear for recovery and skills only. Finish with cornering skills in parking lot.
T	**Key SWIM** 8 × 50 progress by sets of 2 to best effort with 20 sec. rest; 200–400 pull with choice of equipment; 8 × 50 progress to last 4 at best effort; 200–400 pull with choice of equipment; 8 × 50 progress to last 6 at best effort with 30 sec. rest; 200–400 pull with choice of equipment; 8 × 50 best effort with paddles and fins. *Slower swimmers swim 25s in place of 50s.*	**Key RUN Hilly Endurance** Up to 70 min. *Nothing too deep here.* **+ Functional Strength**
W	**RIDE Endurance** 90 min.–3 hr. Initial 30 min. fast rpm, small gear. All focused on posture and pedal stroke. *(Note the effort needs to drop here, as the key sessions are such high load.)* **RUN Off the Bike** 15–25 min. low stress (musculoskeletal load).	**P.M. OFF**
T	**Key SWIM** 3 to 6 rounds of 10 × 50 at 90% effort on the shortest possible send-off; 200 easy recovery at 70% effort	**Key RUN Power** 8 × 2–5 min. Progress 1 to 4 to Z4/5, then last 4 are at best sustained effort. Recover completely with 3–5 min. rest between intervals.
F	**REST DAY** **OR Optional RUN** 30–50 min. shake-out run for the soul. *No real focus here.*	**Optional SWIM** Very low stress, all form-based.
S	**RUN Low Stress** 50–80 min. Z1/2 with the last 2 min. of each 5 min. focused on posture, foot speed, and body position. *Use Tempo Trainer to keep foot speed at lighter effort.* **+ Functional Strength**	**P.M. OFF**
S	**Key SWIM** Up to 56 × 100, swim as 4 to 7 rounds of 3 to 4 × 100 best sustained effort with 30 sec. rest, right into 3 to 4 × 100 buoy easy on 15 sec. rest.	**Key RIDE Endurance** Up to 5 hr. Z2 with Z2/3 on hills, not deep, preferably on road bike. *Focus on form, standing transitions, cornering. This is a foundational ride.* **RUN Off the Bike** 15–40 min. light (musculoskeletal resilience).

SAMPLE TRAINING BLOCK FOR IRONMAN RACE

	WORKOUT 1	WORKOUT 2
M	**RUN** Up to 1 hr. low stress, nothing over Z2. Walk breaks as needed.	**RIDE** Up to 2 hr. very easy, all Z1/2 effort.
T	**Key SWIM** 4 to 6 rounds of 4 × 50 at 90% effort with deck-up (hop out of the pool, stand up, then dive in) following each; right into 300–500 at race effort (80%). **+ Optional RUN** 30–50 min. low stress morning.	**Functional Strength +** **Key RUN Hilly Endurance** 50–70 min. controlled. *Nothing deep today.*
W	**Key Race-Specific RIDE** 1.5–4 hr. In the middle, do 2 × 40–60 min. at race effort, with the last 10 min. just above race effort and +5–10 rpm. Rest 10 min. between intervals. **RUN Off the Bike** 4 × 8 min. at race effort with 2 min. easy between intervals OR *all low stress if focus is on tomorrow.*	P.M. OFF
T	**Key SWIM** 4 × 300, 4 × 250, 4 × 200, 4 × 150, 4 × 100, 4 × 50, all progressing within each set as 70% with 20 sec. rest, 80% with 15 sec. rest, 85–90% with 10 sec. rest, 95% with 5 sec. rest. NO breaks. *Scale as needed.* **+ Functional Strength**	**Race-Specific RUN** Warm up 1 hr. easy pace, Z1/2 to Z2. Then 3 × 20 min. at or just above race pace (Z3) with 2 min. walk between intervals.
F	**RIDE Low Stress** 60–90 min. spin in Z1/2, higher rpm. *Nothing deep today.*	**Optional SWIM** Low stress with no intensity and light pull focus. *Freshen and bridge to tomorrow.*
S	**Key Open-Water SWIM** 9 to 12 × 4–6 min. Swim **set 1** at 75–80%; **set 2** at 80–85% with first and last 100 strokes at take out speed with sighting, **set 3** at full race simulation/ best effort. Repeat progression until done. Rest 90 sec. between sets. *This is the key session this week.*	**RIDE** Warm up 30 min. Z1 at faster rpm; then ride 60 min. endurance Z2 with Z2/3 hills; then 30 min. easy spin Z1, faster rpm to flush out the effort. **OR RUN/RIDE** 50–60 min. low-stress run *followed by* 30 min. easy spin Z1/2 with faster rpm.
S	**Key Race-Specific RIDE** Warm up 30 min., then 4 × 10 min. under race effort Z1/2; 40 min. at race effort Z2/3 to Z3; 10 min. above race effort Z3 to Z3/4. All continuous with no breaks. **RUN** 5 min. light (elites go faster here specific to race plan), 20 min. at race pace, 10 min. at or above race pace.	P.M. OFF

	WORKOUT 1	WORKOUT 2
M	**Optional SWIM** Pull set of 100s, 75s, and 50s all long and easy. *Focus on form and light speed.*	**Optional RIDE** 1–2 hr. at higher rpm and small gear for recovery. *Focus on form and pedal stroke/skills.* Finish with cornering skills in parking lot. **OR RUN** 40–50 min. low stress shake-out. **OR REST** if fatigued.
T	**Key SWIM** 2 to 3 rounds of 5 × 100 best sustained effort with 45 sec. rest; 2 × 50 easy with 20 sec. rest. Rest 30 sec. between rounds. Then swim 300–600 pull at 60%. Then 2 to 3 rounds with paddles and fins as 5 × 50 best effort; 2 × 25 easy with 20 sec. rest. Rest 30 sec. between rounds.	**Key RUN** On hilly or rolling terrain, 3 × 15–25 min. sustained tempo Z3+ effort. Rest 5 min. between intervals. **+ Functional Strength**
W	**Key RIDE Endurance** 90 min.–3 hr. Initial 30 min. fast rpm and small gear. *Focus on posture and pedal stroke. (Note that effort needs to drop here because key sessions are such high load.)* **RUN Off the Bike** 15–25 min. low stress (musculoskeletal load)	**P.M. OFF** **OR SWIM** Low stress and easy.
T	**SWIM** 8 × 300 [or 250, 200, 150] progress effort by sets of 2 from very easy to strong. 300–500 pull at 60%. Repeat progression with half distance: 8 × 150 [125, 100, 75] following same progression; then swim 150–250 pull at 60%. *Set yourself up for success; adjust based on fatigue.*	**Key RIDE** 6 × 10 min. progress every 2 sets to finish very strong effort with great form. Rest 5 min. between intervals. **RUN Off the Bike** 6 × 3–5 min. progress every 2 sets to very strong. Rest 2 min. between intervals.
F	**REST DAY** **Optional RUN** 30–50 min. shake-out for the soul. *No real focus here.*	**Optional SWIM** Very low stress, all form-based.
S	**Key RUN Low Stress** 50–80 min., all Z1/2 with the last 2 min. of each 5 min. focused on posture, foot speed, and body position. *Use Tempo Trainer to keep foot speed lighter.* **+ Functional Strength**	**P.M. OFF**
S	**Key Open-Water SWIM** *Choose a 4–6-min. course.* **Round 1:** 3 loops, progress effort 70%, 80%, 90% with beach exit/entry after each loop. **Round 2:** 1 loop easy, 2 × 2 loops progress effort 80%, 90% with a beach exit. **Round 3:** 1 loop easy, 2 loops best effort with beach exit. Cool down.	**Key Race-Specific RIDE** 3.5–4 hours, with final 60–90 min. at race effort. If possible, end with 3 × 10 min. strong big-gear climb at Z3+. Spin down 5 min. between each interval. **RUN Off the Bike** 20 min. right at race effort to finish.

SAMPLE TRAINING BLOCK FOR HALF-IRONMAN RACE

	WORKOUT 1	WORKOUT 2
M	**RUN Low Stress** Up to 1 hr., nothing over Z2. Walk breaks as needed.	**RIDE Low Stress** Up to 2 hr. all Z1/2, very easy effort.
T	**Key SWIM** 4 to 6 rounds of 3 × 50 at 95% effort with deck-up following each (hop out of the pool, stand up, then dive in) right into 250–400 at 80–85%, close to race effort. **Optional RUN** 30–50 min. easy morning, for resilience.	**Key RUN Endurance** 50–70 min., controlled. *Nothing deep today.* **+ Functional Strength**
W	**Key Race-Specific RIDE** 1.5–3.5 hr. In the middle of the ride, 2 to 3 × 5 min. just under race pace, 3 to 5 × 10 min. right at race pace, 2 to 3 × 5 min. just above race pace. All 5 min. easy spin between intervals. **RUN Off the Bike** 20 min. low stress. Finish with 6 × 10 sec. fast strides with 1–2 min. easy between intervals.	P.M. OFF
T	**Key SWIM** 4 × 300, 4 × 250, 4 × 200, 4 × 150, 4 × 100, 4 × 50 all progressing within each set as 70% with 20 sec. rest, 80% with 15 sec. rest, 85–90% with 10 sec. rest, 95% with 5 sec. rest. No breaks. *Scale as needed for level.* **+ Functional Strength**	**RUN Hilly Endurance** 60–90 min. Gentle building effort as strong as legs feel.
F	**RIDE** 60–90 min. spin, low stress Z1/2 with higher rpm. *Nothing deep here.*	**Optional SWIM** Low stress with no intensity and light pull focus. *Freshen here to bridge to tomorrow.*
S	**Open-Water SWIM** 9 to 12 × 4–6 min., progressing in sets of 3 as 75–80%, 80–85% with 1st and last 100 strokes at takeout speed with sighting, full race-simulation best effort. Rest 90 sec. between intervals. *This is the key session of the week.*	**Key RUN** 6 to 10 × 4–6 min. at 110–115% race pace with 4 min. rest between intervals.
S	**RIDE Hilly Endurance** Up to 4 hr. In the middle include 2 × 15–25 min. at race pace with 15 min. between intervals.	P.M. OFF

WEEK 2

	WORKOUT 1	WORKOUT 2
M	**Optional SWIM** Long and easy pull set of 100s, 75s, and 50s, all form reset and low stress. *All form-based and light speed.*	**Optional RIDE Light** 1–2 hr. all higher rpm, small gear. For recovery and skills only. Finish with cornering skills in parking lot. *Maintain focus on form and pedal stroke.* **OR RUN** 40–50 min. low stress shake-out. **OR REST** if fatigued.
T	**Key SWIM** 3 × 200 progress 1 to 3 to close to best effort (faster than race pace). Then swim 200s at that pace with 1 min. rest. Once you fail to maintain pace, move to 150s with 1 min. rest at SAME pace/100. Once you fail to maintain, move to 100s at the same pace with 1 min. rest. This should total up to 12 swims.	**Key RUN Tempo** On rolling terrain, 2 to 4 × 12–18 min. at strong sustained tempo pace (Z3+), with 5 min. rest between each interval. **+ Functional Strength**
W	**RIDE Endurance** 90 min.–3 hr. Initial 30 min. fast rpm, small gear. *All focus on posture and pedal stroke. Effort needs to drop here as key sessions are high load.* **RUN Off the Bike** 15–25 min. low stress (musculoskeletal load)	**P.M. OFF** **OR SWIM** Light and easy, low stress.
T	**SWIM** 8 × 300 (or 250, 200, 150) progress effort by sets of 2 from very easy to strong; then swim 300–500 pull at 60%. Repeat same progression at half distance: 8 × 150 (125, 100, 75), then 150–250 pull at 60%.	**Key RIDE** 8 to 10 × 4–6 min., progress intervals by sets of 2 to the last 4 to 6 at very strong effort with great form. Rest should equal interval. **RUN Off the Bike** 6 × 3–5 min. progress by sets of 2 to very strong with 2 min. rest between intervals.
F	**REST DAY** **OR Optional RUN** 30–50 min. shake-out for the soul. *No real focus here.*	**Optional SWIM** Very low stress, all form-based.
S	**Key RUN Low Stress** 50–80 min. all Z1/2 with the last 2 min. of each 5 min. focused on posture, foot speed, and body position. *Use Tempo Trainer to keep foot speed at lighter effort.* **+ Functional Strength**	**P.M. OFF**
S	**Open-Water SWIM** *Choose a 4– 6-min. course.* **Round 1:** 3 loops progress effort 70%, 80%, 90% with a beach exit/entry following each loop. **Round 2:** 1 loop easy, 2 × 2 loops progress effort 80%, 90% with a beach exit. **Round 3:** 1 loop easy, 2 loops best effort with beach exit. Cool down.	**Key Race-Specific RIDE** 2.5–3.5 hr. Warm up, then ride 3 to 5 × 20 min. as 15 min. at race pace, 5 min. above race pace with faster rpm with 10 min. rest between each interval.

SAMPLE TRAINING BLOCK FOR OLYMPIC-DISTANCE RACE

	WORKOUT 1	WORKOUT 2
M	**RUN Low Stress** Up to 40 min., nothing over Z2. Walk breaks as needed.	P.M. OFF
T	**Key SWIM** 1 to 3 rounds of 4 × 25 fast with deck-up; 5 to 8 × 100 as best sustainable pace (85%) with 7–10 sec. rest; then 2 × 25 with deck-up, 200–300 easy with buoy between sets.	**Key RUN Endurance** 40–60 min. controlled. *Nothing deep today.* **+ Functional Strength**
W	**Key Race-Specific RIDE** 1.5–2.5 hr. After warm-up, do 3 × 4 min. at 110% race effort, with 4 min. spin between intervals; 2 × 10 min. at 100% race effort with 5 min. rest between intervals; 3 × 2–4 min. at 110% race effort for as long as you can hold the effort with 4 min. rest between intervals. **RUN Off the Bike** 3–5 min. at race effort, then 10–15 min. easy shake-out light.	P.M. OFF
T	**Key SWIM Endurance** 8 × 125–250 progress by sets of 2 to 90% on the last 2, all with 30 sec. rest. **+ Functional Strength**	**Optional RUN Endurance** 30–50 min. low intensity.
F	**Optional SWIM** Low stress with no intensity and light pull focus. *Need to freshen here. A bridge to tomorrow.*	P.M. OFF
S	**Open-Water SWIM** 8 × 3 min. loops, odds easy, evens full race simulation at best effort. Include start, middle, and beach finish, with 2 min. rest between intervals. *This is the key session of the week.*	**Key RUN Tempo** 3 to 5 × 8–12 min. Z3+, with 4 min. rest between intervals.
S	**Key RIDE Hilly Endurance** Up to 3 hr. *Nothing deep today.*	P.M. OFF

	WORKOUT 1	WORKOUT 2
M	**Optional RIDE Light** 1–2 hr. all higher rpm and small gear. For recovery and skills only. Finish with cornering skills in parking lot. *Maintain focus on form and pedal stroke.* **OR RUN** 40–50 min. low stress shake-out. **OR REST** if fatigued.	**P.M. OFF**
T	**Key SWIM Race Simulation** 11 × 150 where 1, 2, 6, 10, and 11 are fast (90–95%); 3 and 7 are 70–75% controlled; 4, 5, 8, and 9 are strong and sustained (85% effort). *Simulates race start, settle, strong, buoy turns, settle, strong and sustained, and strong finish.*	**Key RUN** 8 to 12 × 4 min. as 2 to 3 rounds of 4 × 4 min. at 105–110% race effort, with 4 min. easy between intervals.
W	**RIDE Endurance** 1.5–2 hr. Initial 30 min. at fast rpm, small gear. *All posture and pedal stroke focus. The effort needs to drop here as the key sessions are high load.* **NO RUN.**	**P.M. OFF** **OR SWIM** Light and easy.
T	**SWIM Light Endurance** Pull 20 to 40 × 50 at 80% with every 5th fast, rest only 5–7 sec. between intervals. Then 20 to 40 × 25 with paddles at 80–85%, with every 5th as a sprint, rest only 5–7 sec. between intervals.	**Key RIDE Hilly Endurance** Up to 2 hr. Z3, with bigger gear. **RUN Off the Bike** Following warm-up do 6 × 10 sec. strides with 1–2 min. easy jog between intervals.
F	**REST DAY** **OR Optional RUN** 30–50 min. shake-out run for the soul. *No real focus here.*	**Optional SWIM** Very low stress, all form-based.
S	**Key RUN Low Stress** 40–70 min. all Z1/2 with the last 2 min. of each 5 min. focused on posture, foot speed, and body position. *Use Tempo Trainer to keep foot speed at lighter effort.* **+ Functional Strength**	**P.M. OFF**
S	**Key Open-Water SWIM** 2 to 3 × 8–10 min. full race simulation with 5 min. easy swimming between intervals.	**Key Race-Specific RIDE** 6 × 10 min. at race effort with 5–10 min. easy spinning between intervals. **RUN Off the Bike** 5 min. at race effort with good form, then 15–20 min. easy float.

11

Racing: When Performance Counts

We have spent the vast majority of the book discussing your training and how to properly prepare for, and recover from, hard work. At the end of the day, what really counts is race day. We *prepare* in training so that we can *perform* on race day. I say this with a wry smile on my face. In my career as both an international-level swimmer and a professional triathlete, I could easily have been classified as the world's best trainer. I poured massive effort into my training and could perform at a level well above anything my race performance would indicate, but race day seldom revealed my potential. The harsh truth is that I failed to time my best performances to arrive on race day. As I reflect on my long-past swimming and triathlon careers, there's less emotion and ego to cloud my judgment, but I realize now that my underperformance had little to do with nerves or fear. The truth is that *fitness does not equate with performance.* I was a victim of my own work ethic, which had little logical application and only a passing reference to recovery, nutrition, or other factors that would help me prepare for the big day. I repeatedly turned up on race day overtrained and underperforming, and my career ended as I slumped into fatigue.

Following plenty of self-reflection, I applied these lessons to the careers of other athletes, and I have been lucky to work with athletes who are more talented than I ever was. With this, I have always given special attention to the *process* of training—that is, remaining healthy, balanced, and productive—as well as the run-in to racing that allows performance to come out of the training. This chapter is intended to help you prepare for the big day, from your training run-in to your race-week protocol. Read on, and arrive prepared.

COMPONENTS OF RACE-DAY PERFORMANCE

The conventional approach to tapering for a triathlon has long imitated more traditional sports such as track and field or competitive swimming. It always seemed crazy to me that triathletes would try to implement the taper protocols that are typically used for events lasting 10 seconds to 15 minutes. Endurance sports lasting between 2 and 17 hours demand a very different approach and psychology. I urge athletes to view their race preparation through a lens that better accommodates a sport as complex as triathlon.

Training run-in. This is commonly referred to as a "taper," but I feel that this terminology reinforces all of the misconceptions surrounding the lead-up to race day. Moreover, I would recommend that you truly taper your training only once or twice in a calendar year. That said, the final two or three weeks of training before a major event do require careful consideration in order to achieve the goal of maintaining every ounce of fitness, arriving at race day feeling fresh, and being physiologically prepared to perform close to your potential.

Nutrition and hydration. You should give careful consideration to the approach you will take with your fueling, nutrition, and hydration in the week leading up to a major event, on the morning of the event, and during the event itself. Plenty of mistakes occur in race week as a result of an athlete's aim to do "something special" to gain energy. You will typically find out the hard way that simplicity rules.

Course planning. A smart athlete will have a thorough understanding of what awaits him or her on race day. This means you will need to do your homework on the swim course, the bike course, and the run course. Make a plan for how you will manage the conditions and terrain, and you will create a greater opportunity to showcase your fitness and performance-readiness.

ADVANCE PREPARATION FOR RACING

Planning is critical to racing, as a proper plan can increase predictability and familiarity with what you can expect on race day. Let's take the bike leg, for example. You will need to study the route and elevation profile and check the weather forecast. Pre-riding the course is certainly the best preparation, but if it is not an option, a lot can be achieved in 30 minutes of online research. Also, draw what you can from previous race reports and experiences—what went well and not so well. Beyond this, how was your pacing? How did you run off the bike? What problems did you encounter? This information and many other factors can help you plan for a particular race. What you learn will influence the equipment you choose—tires, wheels, gearing, on-bike hydration system, clothing, etc. Every course demands a different mix of options and presents certain limitations. For example, a fully closed course allows more cornering freedom than one with varying degrees of traffic. Learning how to navigate different terrain safely while constantly monitoring your energy level and apply your pedaling and riding tools—such as proper standing or effective cornering—is an ongoing process for every athlete at every level.

In addition, you should learn about the swim course, including buoy positions, sighting cues, location of the sun, possible currents, and the optimal place to line up at the start. Then, of course, you still need to map transitions and logistics as well as all of the dynamics and terrain of the run portion of the race. What do they say: "Piss-poor planning equals piss-poor performance"?

Tactics. Your racecourse reconnaissance, knowledge of your personal strengths and weaknesses, and even some potential thoughts of your competition (if you are elite) should inform your race plan. All of this homework provides the framework and road map of how you will approach the race. Your task then is to remain focused on the requirements of the day—the process—instead of the result or outcomes.

Equipment. A shocking number of athletes, professionals included, arrive at race day with dirty, ill-prepared equipment. The biggest culprit is the bicycle, with dirty chains, tires with cuts in them, or gears and brakes that are not properly aligned or tuned. If this is you, you are giving away speed and setting yourself up for frustration. I will never forget an amateur triathlete whom we invited to join us at a pro training camp a few years ago. Brian's equipment was by far the best prepared and maintained, and he was a family man running a business of 150 employees. In a playful yet serious way, we used him to shame the pros! Their equipment has been sparkling ever since that day.

Warm-up. This is one of the most ignored elements of triathlon racing. If you ever stand near the transition area before a race, you will notice how amazingly little warm-up many athletes do before a race. This includes, I am afraid, many of the pros. A thorough and appropriate warm-up is a key ingredient to a successful day. We'll address the pre-race warm-up later in the chapter (page 277).

Race execution. The final piece of the puzzle is the actual execution of your race. Your mind-set, thought process, and pacing all factor into how the race plays out for you. We will discuss some of the common mistakes as well as winning mind-sets and strategies to allow your performance to bubble to the surface.

THE RACE RUN-IN

The extent to which you might alter your training as you prepare for an event is dependent on the relative importance of your upcoming race and where you are in your season. Naturally, I will focus mostly on preparation for a major event, or A-race, but let's first consider an early-season race.

Setting Up an Early-Season Race

Not all races are created equal. Early-season races are wonderful opportunities to build fitness, test pacing and fueling strategies, and maintain vibrancy and passion for the sport. View them as what they are: benchmarks of performance. A common mistake is for athletes to over-recover or undertrain going into early-season races. I have a simple rule of thumb: *Rest either up to 3 days or more than 10 days, but never any amount in between.* Most athletes who rest more than 2 to 3 days fall into a feeling of lethargy and fatigue as they recuperate and heal from previous training, which leads to a poor performance. It's not a great way to race.

Run-in to a Secondary Race

4 DAYS OUT	Endurance focus: extended duration at lower intensity
3 DAYS OUT	Final intervals: building efforts on the swim and bike
2 DAYS OUT	Lighter day and recuperation
1 DAY OUT	Race prep sessions
RACE DAY	Thorough warm-up followed by pre-race fuel and hydration—then *race*!

The *gray* days highlight a focus on recuperation and limited stress. The *blue* days highlight a focus on maintaining fitness and preparing, with a little necessary intensity to remain sharp.

If you are following a smart training program that is challenging without accumulating massively irreparable fatigue, you should gain a really positive energy and performance lift from just a few days of recuperation. This is how you should consider approaching a secondary race. During race week you should avoid sessions that create massive muscular damage or stress, such as very long runs or extended intervals at maximal steady-state effort, but the theme of your regular training still applies.

Recovery

While the drop-in to a B-race is shorter, it remains critical to thoroughly recover from the race before resuming heavy-load training. This fact is often ignored by overenthusiastic, highly motivated athletes. Good performances are followed by excited training, while poor performances are followed by a vengeful return to training in order to make amends. Patience is key, and true recovery is a worthy investment to allow a positive return to training, bring about consistency, and avoid injury.

I like athletes to be aware of two main types of fatigue that occur with racing in triathlon. In layman's terms, the first is the muscular damage that occurs, and the second is the hormonal stress that comes with the effort. Muscular damage is easy to spot—you may be hobbling around with sore legs for one to three days after the race. The good news is that muscular damage is quick to repair, but take this with a grain of salt, as it can lead to a false sense of recovery. Have you ever finished an event and within a few days felt great? You eagerly returned to training and felt surprisingly good, but within 7 to 10 days you felt a curtain of fatigue and heaviness descend over every session? This is a sure sign of underrecovery from the race and the hormonal damage that has occurred from racing.

Following a race, you should be prepared to allow yourself a little physical recuperation and a break from the emotional demands of training. Allow your body to lead you as you ramp back up to the full training schedule; recovery can take less or more time than anticipated, depending on various factors for each individual athlete. To cope with this, I encourage athletes to focus on lighter-endurance work, set up any intervals as building or progressive to allow a feeling of success and management, and make smart decisions about their effort level relative to how they feel. It is typically 7 to 10 days after a race before I tell athletes to forget about the B-race and completely move on. (Recovery from an Ironman takes longer, of course, but we don't have too many B-level Ironman races!) This doesn't mean you can expect 7 to 10 days of low-value training, but a high awareness of fatigue level and training management is necessary.

Setting Up an A-Race

I see many athletes miss opportunities to perform well on race day because of mistakes made during the "taper" portion of training. Before we delve into the details, let's consider what a taper is as well as what it isn't. It is well understood that training is an essential stress that should force adaptations that, in turn, allow us to perform better. In other words, we get fitter, stronger, and more powerful. The taper acts as the essential link between the hard training and readiness to perform at, or close to, our best level on a specific day. This should mean that the purpose of a taper, or run-in, is to:

- **Maintain fitness:** Hold on to all cardiovascular and muscular endurance gained through the endurance training.
- **Heighten neuromuscular coordination:** Sharpen fitness to enable optimal dialogue between brain and muscles—motor skills are better with adequate rest.

- **Be emotionally fresh and rested:** Allow enough recuperation to heighten emotional readiness for the grand efforts of race performance.
- **Fine-tune race performance:** Part physical, part emotional, think of the taper as final programming of and familiarity with race-type effort.

As you can see, rest is an important component of a run-in. Your race run-in should not be a desperate attempt to focus on recuperating from the rigors of training. Many athletes employ a "rest and hope" strategy, training very hard until X number of days before the race, then resting in the hope of reaching a fresh state by race day. This undermines confidence because they will inevitably feel flat and fatigued when they begin to rest, and this feeling carries over into race day, by which point they are feeling lethargic, with a loss of fitness. For this reason, I like athletes to rest early and to undergo a *pre-run-in "clean-out"* two to three weeks before race day to rid them of the deep residual fatigue that is often associated with heavy training. This will leave the athlete feeling a little dormant initially, but there is still time to focus on sharpening and a run-in to the race that is familiar because it includes some "real" training.

The run-in to an A-race is relatively different from a taper for a shorter event, but it works well because the *relative intensity* of triathlon is much lower. Triathlon is a true endurance sport, which can be beneficial to its athletes and

Run-in to an A-Race

10 DAYS OUT	Include some very strong building efforts at or around threshold in swim and/or bike
7 DAYS OUT	Hit race-specific intensity or a minisimulation on the same day of the week as race day
3–4 DAYS OUT	Touch intensity for the last time, fit in a final endurance-based session (not on the same day)
2 DAYS OUT	Typically the day to "clean out"—truly rest and recuperate
1 DAY OUT	Light training with some smooth building efforts. Don't be afraid of a little work. I often ask athletes to ride until they "feel good." This might be 20 minutes, or it might take 100 minutes.

Make fueling a priority throughout the race run-in—it's absolutely critical to support the lighter training load. Follow every session with the appropriate fueling protocol.

TYPICAL RACE RUN-IN

TRAINING BLOCK	6–12 weeks race-specific preparation.
CLEAN OUT	2–3 weeks prior to the A-event, including 3–5 days of very low stress and recuperation. As the body responds to the rest, some lethargy and heaviness will be felt.
RUN-IN	A mini-build of regular training, but at a reduced intensity and load. The goal is a familiar pattern of training, avoiding any sessions that create deep fatigue. Key sessions are mostly focused around race-specific intensity and simulation.
RACE PREPARATION	2 to 3 days prior to the race is the time to clean out and truly freshen up in order to avoid feeling dormant on race day.

RACE DAY

If you are still feeling fatigued in the final 7 to 14 days before a race, you are authorized to inject more rest into the final stretch. Conversely, if you are feeling very fresh, you can maintain your rhythm and work with a little added endurance training.

coaches. The longer the duration of the event, the less we need to perfect the day of performance. Endurance athletes have more time to find their rhythm and get their "engines" really turning over, so they have greater leeway in exact readiness. It is one of the reasons many triathletes love to have weekly templates of training, with repetition built into the program.

Don't let anyone tell you there is only one way to go about the final weeks of training. The point is to create habits and an approach that are familiar and *make you feel good.* I deploy the run-in I've described here with almost every athlete I work with, but as we delve into the details of daily prescription, there is a wide array of possibilities. The final two weeks of Meredith Kessler's Ironman preparation look entirely different from Jesse Thomas's half-Ironman preparation. I have never seen a run-in like Meredith's, which includes no riding in the final two days, 4 × 800 of swimming two days prior, and a 20- to

30-minute run at 4 a.m. on race morning! As you develop in your sport and get the opportunity to learn from consistent racing, you will begin to refine the approach that works for you, so be a student of your own sport and readiness.

A couple of years ago I was reminded of how different race preparation can be for different athletes. In addition to being one of the sport's great ambassadors, Meredith Kessler is a very caring person. As a coach, I felt that she was a little *too* caring—she was spending too much energy and emotional capacity thinking of others in her approach to racing. She was e-mailing every amateur she knew prior to races to wish them luck; she was invested in whether her friends and family had comfortable accommodations when coming to watch her race; and she was more than willing to give her time or equipment to those who had forgotten or broken theirs. Traditional thought would dictate that, as a professional, she should be "effectively selfish" in her race lead-up and put her well-intentioned, loving habits on pause. I asked her to set up an "out of office" reply on her e-mail, stop giving to others during race week, and save her energy. It was a battle. I came to realize that my intervention was taking away something that actually energizes her. In many ways, helping and supporting others provides Meredith with passion for her own racing. It was a mistake to pull her away from who she *is*. We don't do it anymore, and Meredith continues to help others and love race week. We do ensure that she also maintains enough rest and recovery to allow each race to be a positive experience.

Testing Your Approach to Race Preparation

It will take some trial and error to refine your race preparation. Learn what works for you, not others, and be honest and systematic with your approach. Aim to establish good habits in training that you can carry into race week. Here's a recap to guide your run-in to any race.

Limit the taper. Big endurance events don't require a long taper. If you train smart, stay healthy, and don't carry too much fatigue, solid performances can arrive out of only a few days of recuperation or rest.

Rest early, then sharpen. Rest and heal a few weeks before a race then sharpen going into a race with a mini-block of training that is familiar to regular training but is designed so as not to create big fatigue. A couple of light days prior to the race will adequately open up performance.

Do building intervals. In the final 10 to 14 days all intervals are created as building intensity in order to provide more control of effort. Also, this is not the time to try to find confidence through "validation" efforts. How you feel is not critical to your upcoming performance, so never go above the prescribed intensity just to build confidence.

Hit it the day before. Some athletes perform best on the second day of hard work. I have had athletes ride two hours with progressive intervals the day prior to an Ironman victory. If you often feel flat or lethargic while racing, you might add a little duration to your training the day prior to the race.

Really rest. In direct contrast, you might respond really well to big rest. Often my most resilient trainers like big rest. I have some athletes who only complete a 20-minute swim in the final two days prior to racing. They seldom have issues getting their engines going, whereas others would really suffer. Test it out!

Be open to warm-up. You need to warm up before you race, but how much? Some require plenty of work. Meredith Kessler includes a 30-minute easy run 3 hours prior to a race start, but I promise you that Jesse Thomas is still asleep! It all depends on the individual.

Let the body drive, not the mind. Don't force anything in race week. Let your body drive the efforts, and ensure that you never chase speed, effort, or power. If you feel lethargic, don't push yourself; if you feel fresh, bottle it for race day. The more you let your body drive things (and the less you judge yourself), the more your body and mind will give you on race day.

RACE-WEEK NUTRITION AND HYDRATION

As you progress through your race preparation, it is very easy to be drawn into making major changes in your eating and fueling. Because you are likely to have more time on your hands due to the reduced training load, and you naturally have a strong desire to do everything right, nutrition is an area that tends to receive special focus. Many athletes start packing vitamins, eating extremely clean diets, and either loading up on or restricting calories to either build energy reserves or avoid adding any unwanted pounds. None of these strategies have a positive influence on your performance. The good news is that race-week nutrition should be relatively simple—there is no need to alter much. You don't need to go on a crazy diet, and you certainly shouldn't restrict or pile on the calories.

Eat your normal diet. Maintain your regular diet in terms of quantity, quality, and timing. There is just one adjustment I would recommend, especially if you have experienced gastrointestinal issues on race day—avoid eating too many leafy greens and vegetables in the final 48 hours. You do want to ensure that you have complete energy stores, but if you maintain the quantity of consumption while reducing the training load, this will not be a problem. Of course I hope that the quality of your regular diet is relatively good in the first place!

Focus on fueling. While this is always appropriate, pay special attention to fueling during and especially after your training sessions. With sessions being lighter, many tend to forget to fuel, but we want to ensure that your reserves are replenished.

Daily hydration. Maintain regular and consistent daily hydration with water, but add a little sodium and citrus juice to each glass, and consider a hydration solution with a similar mix in the final 2 to 3 days prior to the race. Avoid consuming massive amounts of water throughout the day.

Avoid most supplements. In the final couple of weeks prior to race day, it may be beneficial to take a simple calcium-magnesium (Ca-Mg) supplement prior to bed. Magnesium gets depleted with heavy training, and it is a key component of muscle contraction. This simple addition may stave off race-day cramps. Beyond Ca-Mg, there is little to no benefit to adding vitamins, minerals, or other supplements. Anything that truly works is more than likely to contain something it shouldn't. Don't fall for the hype.

Consume protein before bed. Maximize recovery and protein synthesis while you sleep by consuming 15 to 20 grams of protein immediately before bed.

Drink a beer. Come on, it is only a race. Have a beer with dinner if you want one. It won't hurt.

RACE MORNING

We now arrive at race morning, and it is time to fuel up and prepare for the race itself. If you have been appropriately fueling and hydrating in the days and weeks leading up to the event, your muscles should be full of glycogen (the stored form of carbohydrate), and the additional calories you eat will simply be a top-off of immediate fuel and calories. Remember that you cannot store calories in the way a camel stores water, and you don't need to start a race feeling bloated and full. Let's explore a simple race-day process that might help you arrive at the line ready to perform.

Before Leaving for the Race

I recommend waking several hours before the gun goes off. This will ensure that your body has time to synthesize the calories you consume. I prefer to first eat a small amount of protein in order to suppress elevated cortisol from sleep, then do a light, short run. Breakfast can be light, with a focus on protein, good oils, and some carbohydrate. As you can see, carbohydrate doesn't need to be the focus of the meal. Don't avoid coffee; a cup to get you going is fine by me.

Race morning can be confusing, so help clear your mind by having a checklist of all that you need to accomplish as well as everything you need to have with you. This might include body marking, special-needs drop-off, wetsuit, goggles, visor or hat, water bottles, and everything else you can imagine. Read through the checklist before you leave for the race to ensure that you have everything you need.

Setup & Prep

You are now ready to execute the checklist: setting up or checking your bike; ensuring that you are wearing the correct gear; dropping off any necessary materials; and completing a review of the transition flow, exits, sunrise time, and swim conditions. All of this should be completed at least 30 minutes prior to the start. This means you need to plan your arrival at the transition area accordingly. Here are the five aspects of your setup that require your attention before you begin to warm up.

- **Race essentials:** Complete all aspects required by the race—body marking, timing chip, special needs, etc.

- **Route:** Check transition and course routes to ensure that you know your path.
- **Conditions:** Take note of water conditions, sun, wind, and any other environmental factors.
- **Equipment:** Make sure your equipment is ready by checking tire pressure, gears (yes, check them in the morning), transition setup, brakes (are they rubbing?), etc.
- **Fuel:** Ensure that hydration and fuel are set up for the bike and ready for the run.

Pre-Race Warm-up

I see many triathletes simply kiss their friends good-bye and then hop in the water and hit the initial few hundred meters at a close-to-max output. Not the best way to start a long day. The warm-up is the most ignored piece of triathlon racing. I'm not talking about a few arm swings and two minutes of easy swimming.

Think about the part of your training session when you typically feel that you are at your best—it certainly isn't the warm-up. It's no different on race day—you need an easy warm-up and then a short pre–main set to open the engine and prepare the body for race effort. A proper warm-up is not a waste of calories; it is essential to allow performance.

I like my athletes to complete a 20- to 30-minute pre-race warm-up session, assuming it is manageable. The first portion of the warm-up should focus on mobility, with some dynamic exercises. Following this, I like athletes to raise their core temperature. This typically includes a 10- to 15-minute light jog. In cold conditions, you might opt to run in your wetsuit—just enough to get the metabolism rolling. The final portion is the swim warm-up. If the water is warm, or warm enough, then you should absolutely plan on an extended 10- to 15-minute swim warm-up that includes easy swimming, gradual building efforts, and then a few "easy-speed" sprints to wake up the neuromuscular system. Of course, this is not always possible, but make every attempt to do it. If the water is particularly cold, prolonged exposure to it won't be beneficial. In this case you can rely on using bands on dry land or even simply arm swings. Use your best judgment.

You are now ready to go, and it is all about the process and execution. Sounds pretty simple, doesn't it?

RACING MIND-SET

There are plenty of excellent books on sports psychology, although many athletes dismiss this subject and assume that mind-set doesn't require consideration. However, mind-set and psychology are the next area of great performance breakout—mark my words. Here I will simply touch on my recommendations for how to approach your racing emotionally and provide a framework for your race plan. As with everything, you can execute a plan only if you have a plan in the first place, so ensure that you think about this as you read on.

Think About Process, Not Outcome

At purplepatch, we talk about *process, not outcome.* We get out of bed for early-morning sessions with a deep desire to improve. When it is cold and rainy, our dreams and goals can help us through the tough sessions. They help with motivation and follow-through. Whether your goal is finishing, qualifying for Kona, getting on the podium, or beating last year's results, put it toward the back of your mind on race day. These are *outcomes*, and you need to focus on the *journey toward these outcomes* when you actually race. Once the gun goes off, almost your entire focus is on your individual task list of process and execution as well as smart reaction to the dynamic environment of racing. The furthest thing from your mind, at least until you are going through some tough times and need a pick-me-up to drive on, should be your hoped-for outcomes. You should also aim to avoid self-evaluation on how the race is progressing, predictions, or time-chasing while you are on the course. Whether it is form, fueling, pacing, or course management, your biggest success will come from executing one step at a time without looking too far forward or back as you remain in the moment. This sounds simple but requires practice and confidence.

Narrow Your Focus

You will have a stronger mind-set if your focus is on you—the individual—not your competition. This is especially important as you define your race plan. I like to set out a race plan as a series of tasks to execute. For elite athletes, this means setting out an individual race plan as the primary priority, then considering the race dynamics that occur around them as a secondary task. For amateurs, purely individual tasks are nearly always the only priority. A great common example of something "externally" driven is the swim start. I often hear that the race plan at the swim start is to "find X person's feet, then draft." With this approach, the very first action taken on race day is to make your race execution dependent on someone else. Except in rare cases, I much prefer the swim start task to be driven by effort, line-up, and sighting. Execute an appropriate effort with proper form, ensure that you are swimming the right line, and *then* look to see what is occurring around you and determine whether it is appropriate to join a group or another swimmer. These tasks, driven by effort and strategy, continue all the way through the swim, transition one, the bike, transition two, and then the run. Your race plan doesn't need to be a laundry list of highly detailed projects, but it does have to guide the route from start to finish and prevent you from judging yourself or your performance before you have crossed the line.

It is important that you are aware of what is going on around you without getting distracted. Your number-one priority is execution of your plan, and it is only after you become highly experienced and fully developed as a triathlete that you can and should respond to other athletes' actions or begin to impose yourself on other competitors. For most, the key is to not be sidetracked. For example, on the bike, there is little or no reason to ever look over your shoulder. The only reasonable time to do so is when you are pulling out or have to move laterally, but in essence, the only factors that are important to your race is what you are doing and what is going on in front of you. If you are effectively deploying your effort and energy on the course and executing a well-planned ride, anything that is happening in the rear is only a distraction. In drafting races, assessing the tactical situation behind you should be conscious and planned.

Turn Big Problems into Little Projects

An additional tool to draw on throughout a race is the ability to break down seemingly grand problems into little projects. This is different from the task-driven mentality that should be applied to executing a race plan because it targets the big-picture issues that crop up. As the race progresses, fatigue and pain can accumulate, and this feeling often begins to make our goals dissipate—actually, this effect is as much hormonal as it is mental weakness. How can we keep our heads in the game?

If you have ever read about training for U.S. Navy SEALs or other elite military units, you are probably familiar with the advice that is given to those entering basic training: "Don't look ahead; simply focus on the task at hand." Sounds like process, right? Well, the same applies in endurance sports. When you get into trouble—whether it is fatigue, loss of motivation, or GI distress—don't get drawn into focusing on how far you have left to go. Instead, break the big problem into smaller goals. This might mean breaking a half-marathon run down into 13 × 1-mile mini-intervals or, as Meredith Kessler did in the 2013 Hawaii Ironman, run signpost to signpost before resetting the mind and repeating the process. The more you can use whatever trick helps you forget the big problem and remain focused *in the now*, the better the *result* will be.

PACING

At this point of the book, it would be easy to diverge from the theme of the writing and outline a comprehensive, metrics-driven approach to guiding your race through leveraging the power meter on the bike and the GPS on the run. However, I am going to avoid any details of a metrics-driven approach because it is not the intention of this book and would only send you down a rabbit hole of data. While power meters and GPS can be highly valuable for athletes on race day and are especially useful in training, I don't want athletes to be overly focused on metrics during a race. To be clear, many of my athletes absolutely utilize metrics during racing, but none of my athletes is governed by the practice. Even with all of the technology we have access to, I still believe that race dynamics and your internal clock should act as the primary resources throughout almost every event. Data and metrics are there as high-value feedback, a potential governing force, and a framework for self-assessment and review. There are many comprehensive resources dedicated to the subject of pacing and metrics, so I'll restrict my discussion of pacing to the body (sense of feel) and the mind.

In setting up your approach to race day your pacing of the event and of each of the three disciplines must *reflect your preparation*. In other words, your approach should be similar to that of your training and key sessions. If, for example, you tend to focus on long endurance sessions in much of your training, and your swims revolve around accumulating distance over fast intervals, it would be silly to begin the swim portion at a very high intensity. You are simply not *prepared* to swim at high intensity at the start of a race. Still, most people do this! You can begin aggressively in any portion of the race, or deploy surges of effort on hills or in tailwinds, only if you are prepared to do so. Simply put, racing is a reflection of your training preparation. I encourage the vast majority of my athletes to approach their races as a series of building efforts. Ironically, there is some interesting research under way that seems to indicate that it *may* be preferable to approach racing with a slightly more aggressive approach in the early stages of the time trial, but thus far the research is too limited (focused on short-duration time trials) to cause a shift in current thinking. That said, it is always worthwhile to listen, watch, and learn, so watch this topic for more developments.

Whether competing in Olympic-distance or Ironman-distance events, I like athletes to focus on the middle to end of each discipline and of the overall race. This is called a "negative split"—meaning that you effectively manage the early part of each discipline and then increase effort as the duration continues. The net result should be an even pace throughout, with your best swimming, biking, or running occurring in the middle to end. The specifics of this approach are highly individual, and what I outline here doesn't take into account critical tactics that come into play in elite racing, but it serves as a starting framework for pacing.

Pacing the Race Start

No other discipline in triathlon requires as much specific preparation to build familiarity as the swim portion, yet this preparation is omitted by many athletes. Simulations and race-specific training hold much of the secret to swim success.

This is the part of the swim where many athletes struggle. A mixture of fear, claustrophobia, and panic, the race start induces high emotional stress and great physical cost without much actual progression. Unless you are a front-of-the-pack swimmer or you have the ability to swim most competitors off your feet, you will want to avoid being in the middle of the pack or on the frontline of the swim. I always recommend lining up toward the outside of the start line, typically on the side that allows you to breathe on your favorite side and see the group on that side of you (e.g., if you breathe on the right side, then line up to the far left as you face out toward the swim course). Choose a seeding appropriate to your swimming level: If you are a 1-hour 30-minute Ironman swimmer, don't be at the front of the line or you will find yourself in a turbulent washing machine with competitors swimming over you!

When the gun goes off to signal the race start, the typical reaction is a mad sprint, with most athletes hitting close-to-max effort in the initial 100 meters. There is little to be gained from this tactic, and unless you've specifically trained for the effort, it will come at great cost. *Think about effort, not speed.* At race start you will already be excited and amped up. I encourage you to start at no more than an 80 percent effort, keeping it smooth and controlled. This may sound too easy, and you may worry about "losing feet," but remember that I said *effort*. The vast majority of swimmers, operating at 80 percent effort at a race start, will be swimming very close to the same speed as at 95 percent effort, including rushing and spinning arms. Only the most elite and experienced swimmers can truly hit the top end and still settle into full race effort. Those who begin with a sprint typically fall back to where you are within the first 200 meters as you continue to build your speed without duress. What an energy saving that ends up being—all the while traveling at the same speed! If you are a weaker or less confident swimmer, I suggest avoiding the craziness completely. You will benefit from simply waiting 10 or 15 seconds poststart, then beginning with a nice smooth and relaxed 70 percent effort. Build effort and speed as you progress, and avoid the anarchy and turmoil that occur at many race starts.

Pacing the Swim

Upper- to Upper-Middle-Pack Swimmers

If you are in the top one-third of your wave or the field, it is likely important that you be prepared, physically and emotionally, to swim fast at the start of the race. Notice that I didn't say "hard"—this difference is key. Under high stress, such as in a race start, effort is not always the same thing as speed. I like to teach athletes to be in control—focused on fluid swimming—but to train themselves to swim for a short duration (1 to 4 minutes) at a higher speed without too much cost. This combination takes training and familiarity. It will still hurt, but you can maintain a fluid stroke and fall into real race pace. Beyond this, the swim is a building effort, with particular focus given to buoy turns (in and out), positioning as you head toward the finish, and the goal of never being more than one body length behind the lead swimmer in your group (if you happen to be in one). This means you are ideally the second swimmer.

Middle- to Lower-Level Swimmers

If you are not in the top third of the pack, I suggest avoiding the high-cost surge and effort of early race speed. Instead, begin on the outside of your pack, allow the initial surge to go, then complete a smooth and fluid start to your race. From here, build your effort by a third of the distance, with your best swimming reserved for the middle and final third. You will minimize cost, reduce the risk of getting swept into other swimmers, and open the door for controlled pacing. Why expend energy that you will need later in the race? Most weaker swimmers have vastly more enjoyable and comfortable experiences, not to mention faster swim splits, if they employ this conservative approach.

Pacing the Bike

Much of the approach to the bike can be influenced by the length of the race, terrain, conditions, and individual aspirations, but we can create a general framework for pacing by breaking the ride into quarters.

The initial quarter of the ride is about transitioning from the swim—letting your legs "come to you" and finding rhythm. By this, I mean that in the initial stages of the bike, your focus should be on creating good pedaling while riding one gear lighter than you will for the "meat" of the bike leg and establishing fantastic posture and style. Once you have accomplished these things and found your rhythm, you can begin to build into full race mode. Unfortunately, most triathletes will overexert themselves in the initial stages of the bike. Unless you are a pro with a specific race tactic or need to drive high effort early in the race, I prefer a more cautious approach.

The middle two quarters of the race call for a controlled, even effort. The word to focus on here is "sustainable." Of course, what constitutes a sustainable effort on the bike portion of an Olympic-distance event will be much different than what is needed for an Ironman and its subsequent marathon. Tailored to your event, this is the golden mean that exudes the need for control, patience, and moderation. It is only in the final quarter that increasing effort and focus will likely be required to maintain speed. Remember that, as mentioned in Chapter 7, I like to see riders shift the load on their bodies and stretch the lower back and hips. Gearing up and transitioning out of the saddle, then stretching the lower back and pushing the hips forward is an investment in your readiness to run.

TIPS FOR FASTER RIDING THROUGHOUT THE COURSE

Suppose your training partner rides a similar bike with a similar setup, is the same weight as you, and has the same average power but finishes the course 7 minutes faster. Much of what follows begins to explain how such advantages take shape. Safety is the overriding concern, but it's likely there are strategies you can employ to improve your speed.

- Ride the smoothest piece of road available to you—this is often the right-hand wheel mark of the cars.
- Avoid riding on the shoulder of the road when possible. The greatest risk of puncture lies here because of road debris and broken glass swept aside by traffic, rain or snow, and maintenance equipment.
- Ride a straight line from where you are to where you want to be. Follow the inside radius or make straight lines from the inside of one corner to the inside of the next one. If you need to set up wide for the next corner, head straight there. Shorten the course— there may be hundreds of yards to be saved. (Be aware of possible blocking penalties if you have a lot of competitor traffic around you.)
- Assess the camber. If an uphill corner has steep banking on the inside line, your load will significantly increase. Ride a wider line.
- Find shelter from the headwind. For example, riding closer to the tree line or even a wall (if the road is narrow) can lessen the effect of the wind.
- Most importantly, don't forget to apply everything you have learned about pedaling technique, riding tools, and management of your physical resources.

Too many athletes drift in effort and pace in the final quarter, either as a result of an early effort or because they are prematurely shifting their mind-set to the run. I prefer to wait until the final 10 to 15 km of the riding leg (3 to 4 km for Olympic distance) to turn the focus to the run ahead. At this point, shift up a gear to put slightly less tension on the chain, and begin to focus on the transition process, preparing the body to move from time trial position into running with a series of standing stretches on the bike.

Pacing the Run

Run pacing typically mimics the same pattern as the bike: Effort and speed are managed over four quarters, the first of which begins with the last few kilometers of the bike. In my mind, this marks the start of the run. Proper preparation and mind-set here will assist in the transition to optimal running form. In addition, focus should be given to the initial mile or so of any run leg. Rather than focusing on effort, I prefer that athletes focus on key cues that can assist in run form: Run tall, maintain a forward lean, remain supple, and keep quick feet. These are examples of form-based running cues that can help you find good running more quickly.

Once you find rhythm and form, you can begin to build up your effort to a strong and sustained rhythm. The middle two quarters of the run are more about rhythm and sustained effort. Of course, this doesn't make it easy, but you should not be losing pace or form in this part of the race.

The time to release the hounds and truly chase a strong finish is the final quarter. Pacing can go out the window, and if there is a time for risk, it is now. Ironically, if you have the capacity to increase your effort and pace at this stage of the race, you have likely nailed your efforts. It takes plenty of courage and wisdom to facilitate this type of feeling.

Of course, you are still in a race, and the amount of risk that you take in a race should be determined by the effectiveness and type of training you have completed. For the most part, racing is an expression of the training you have done. This doesn't mean that the hardest trainer will win. In fact, it is the well-trained and well-prepared athlete who can execute a great pacing and race strategy, coupled with a little luck, and pull off a win.

Not every race is going to be perfect, and I have seen athletes finish a race without having achieved the performance that they deserve. However, I have seen many of the same athletes use these struggles as opportunities to learn and evolve, and they have converted them into later winning performances.

As they say, racing is an expression of your preparation. I love this thought because I believe strongly in proper preparation and its ability to instill great confidence in my athletes' performances. I believe the same thing can happen for you!

TROUBLESHOOTING COMMON RACE-DAY PROBLEMS

It is critical to realize that no race is likely to go flawlessly. Triathlon is a dynamic sport with plenty of logistics and a strong reliance on equipment. How you approach obstacles will determine your resilience and overall success. A solutions-based approach is the absolute secret to consistency of performance.

Mechanical issues on the bike. Preparation for these situations starts before race day. Understand how your bike works, and know how to fix a flat tire or a dropped chain. When something happens, don't panic or try to rush the correction. Don't alter your pacing—the distance and duration remain, so stay calm.

Dropped fuel/hydration. The best-laid fueling plans can be destroyed by a dropped water bottle or fuel. Be flexible, and know your *next-best options* from the selection on course. It is always worth doing some training on course fuel and hydration so that nothing is a surprise.

Loss of energy, motivation, mood. It is not uncommon for athletes to experience a sudden negative shift in mood or motivation. This is nearly always *related to calories*. Don't hesitate to reach for additional calories, and quick!

GI distress. Longer-distance endurance athletes often complain of bloating in the run portion of the event. This is normally due to poor pacing, with too high an effort early in the race or too high a concentration of calories relative to hydration. Understand that in this situation, your absorption of calories is greatly compromised. You have two options. The first is to transition to a *very*-low-carbohydrate solution for 15 to 20 minutes, with the aim of stimulating absorption; the second is to eject the contents of your stomach onto the racecourse. I am afraid the second option is the quickest solution. You can then resume fueling with a more diluted approach to your calories, although you may consider transitioning to Coca-Cola as the major fuel source.

Cramps. This might be the least-understood element of endurance performance. Contrary to popular belief, cramps don't likely occur because of sodium loss or dehydration. Instead, they occur because of fatiguing or overused muscles, often from poor bike posture, position, or pacing. You may also have a predisposition to cramping if you arrive with depleted electrolytes and minerals, but don't simply consider lack of sodium to be the culprit. I have seen more athletes benefit from a calcium-magnesium supplement than from a high-load sodium tablet during racing. That said, in the real world, athletes have a highly variable response to mineral and electrolyte replenishment, and it is an area of key trial and error for every athlete. One thing I *don't* comprehend is a high dose of electrolyte pills throughout s race. It defies all we know about muscle contraction and cramping, so I don't condone it.

EPILOGUE

When I met Meredith Kessler, she was a keen amateur Ironman athlete. In fact, she had already completed 20 Ironman races, with her best performance being 11 hours 28 minutes. Although she hadn't yet set the world on fire, she did have consistency, with her last 15 Ironman race times all within a 10-minute spread. Meredith came to me with a simple request: She wanted me to "make her good." Just how good she could be was certainly an unanswerable question on day one, but when I took her for an initial bike ride, I noticed a few things, including great grit and determination ("gumption" has become our buzzword for Meredith over the last five-plus years), enthusiasm, a big engine, and a startling lack of skills. This all added up to an unpolished diamond.

Over the next 12 months, Meredith progressed from an 11.5-hour Ironman to 9 hours 48 minutes. Within two years, she won Ironman Canada. She has become one of the leading Ironman athletes in the world, with six championships to her name so far. What was the recipe? You might think it was a big increase in training load to build her fitness, but it was quite the opposite. General fitness was not a limiter for Meredith. In fact, on reviewing her training program, I was struck by how much training she was accumulating during a week. What also emerged from the review was that most of this training was completed at a very similar intensity, and there was little regard for rest and recovery. She trained, and trained a lot, but was consistently fatigued throughout the process.

The process with Meredith was to take a longer-term view of her progression, and I set up a five-plus-year road map that we followed. The plan included a pretty dramatic drop in volume of weekly training over the initial two years. The goal was to teach her the value of lighter sessions, recovery, and blocks of recuperation. I also wanted to evolve the range of intensities at which she could operate—fitness was already there, but she simply couldn't go "fast." Her power for an Ironman race was the same as for a half-Ironman, which was the same as for Olympic distance. I decided to integrate two to three lighter days each week, hence forcing reduced volume; do barely enough extended-duration training to prepare her for Ironman distance; and focus on increasing intensity and overall power potential. The thought was to "live off" the foundational endurance she had created over the previous seasons.

The results were immediate and dramatic, and Meredith has since gone on to develop a full range of "gears," even showing the potential to be a very good Olympic-distance and half-Ironman athlete. Of course, the approach has to evolve, and after speed and power were developed, we began to refocus on more classic Ironman training. Meredith's journey is not complete, and we still have much to achieve and improvements to make, but we will chase her goals with ongoing specificity and purpose and never forget the importance of recovery along the way.

Working with a Coach

You might be thinking of getting a coach to help you on your path to performance. This is not an easy decision and requires thought and consideration. There is no shortage of triathlon coaches, but you must find one who is the right fit for you. We all have different personalities, needs, and approaches. I have turned down world-class athletes, not because I didn't like them but because I felt I was not the best coach for them. Take time to evaluate the approach a coach takes to training, talk to some of their athletes, and find more than one option. When buying a car, you don't simply buy the first one you see. Instead, you test-drive a few, look at the reviews, and choose one that fits your needs. Do the same with a coach.

The real issue is filtering the good coaches from the bad so that you can begin a journey toward improved performance both in this season and those to come. I have spent a great deal of time thinking about what makes a good coach. At any level of competition, athletes are typically successful if they have access to a smart training plan, education, guidance, and a sense of community. While a smart training plan is the cornerstone of any coaching program, it shouldn't stop there. Every good training plan should include a long-term vision for the athlete, a seasonal road map for training progression, and ongoing review of this progression. The actual daily training plan should facilitate consistent application of training load and a smart progression throughout the racing season. This plan also needs to be flexible and specific enough to allow training to be integrated into an athlete's life and create positive adaptations. A good coach can simplify this part of the process for you.

Coaching is as much about mentoring and tutoring as it is about planning and workouts, and this is where ongoing education enters in. Athletes need to be armed with the knowledge and tools to allow them to evolve their "athletic IQ" and begin to make their own intelligent decisions. This is a never-ending process of guidance for all aspects of performance, including season planning, nutrition, skills, mental approaches, race strategy, sleep, and travel. The list is endless. If a coach is committed to educating you as an athlete and explaining important decisions, you will become smarter and more self-sufficient regarding the supporting components of performance.

A well-laid plan and all the education in the world don't automatically create great athletes. Ongoing feedback, support, guidance, and mentorship are integral to helping you learn along the way, make good decisions, and apply the training plan as intended. This is the toughest part for athletes who are self-coached. Without a strong mentor or guide who can maintain an objective point of view and help make smart decisions, it is challenging to create an ongoing successful career. Athletes need mentors and support, and a good coach can fill that important role.

The final element athletes need to be successful is somewhat of an X-factor. For many athletes, community is a powerful influence that can help accelerate their progression. Few can live in a bubble and thrive. Whether it is being part of a club or a swim program or simply having training buddies, a sense of belonging creates accountability, enjoyment, reward, and support. "Suffer together, succeed together" should be the mantra.

If you are reflecting on your progression as an athlete or thinking about seeking outside advice or guidance, you should consider these elements as you look for a successful setup for yourself. There is little doubt that the optimal coaching environment includes daily interaction and "on-deck" guidance. In San Francisco, we have a series of daily swim, bike, and run sessions for our training group, and much can be gained by the local athletes from the daily interaction, feedback, and guidance. However, many of my elite athletes are dispersed around the world, which makes communication all the more important. For the elite athletes, we bridge the periods of separation with frequent training camps to allow real-life coaching to occur. For amateur athletes, it is not always possible to find a high-quality coach close to home, so they might need to make small compromises in order to support a successful long-distance relationship.

What makes a good coach? The easy answer would be someone who creates champions, but I am not sure I agree with such a simple reply. I will draw from examples of more elite coaches as we explore this question, but the lessons apply to coaches working with athletes at any level. Great coaches succeed in the following areas.

Making "champions." If a coach leads a group of 25 athletes in their careers, and one of these athletes has massive success, but the other 24 experience injury, deep fatigue, short careers, and destruction, is that person a great coach? Did he or she make a champion or destroy many other potential champions? I think it is important to look beyond the results of any single athlete for the trends and history of all the athletes who have worked with an individual coach.

The art of development. True coaching includes taking an athlete with potential and developing them to excellence throughout a career. This journey is complex and shows the coach's ability to not only provide a plan but create vision and a career road map, be a strong teacher and mentor, and empower athletes to succeed. Most coaches agree that stories of development are the ones that provide the biggest source of pride and satisfaction.

Range of assistance. While some coaches have, understandably, types of athletes in which they specialize, great coaches have the ability to lead, develop, and improve a wide range of athletes. This range is less about gender or race distance and more about being dynamic in leading different personalities or body types and athletes who respond to different training approaches in different manners. A one-size-fits-all approach seldom leads to a great coach; rather, it often leads to "one size fits some, and the others fall to the side."

Sharing. This area is another X-factor, but I think it deserves inclusion. Any coach who is willing to open the book of their coaching approach is one who is confident and has thought through their approach and reasoning. For me, it is a sign of confidence and should be embraced by more coaches. There are exceptions, but many coaches who cling to secrecy or refuse to share their methods often lack confidence in what they are doing, or perhaps even in the substance and understanding of what they are prescribing. Good coaches understand that coaching success is not about the workouts. Sure, workout design is important, but a good coach could give a year's worth of workouts to any hopeful, and the chances of the hopeful achieving the same results as any other athlete would be slim. It is the overall recipe, and the execution of that recipe, that makes a coach or program successful.

On a personal note, there are many prominent coaches with whom I would love to discuss coaching methodology and understand their process: Darren Smith, Joel Filliol, Michael Kreuger, Paul Newsome, Brett Sutton, Lubos Bilek, Phil Skiba, Dan Lorang, Clif English, Siri Lindley, Neal Henderson, and many more. Some of these peers I already know, and some I don't. We may not see eye to eye on everything—in fact, we may approach performance in a very different way—but I know that conversations with those who are successful in the sport help me continue to evolve as a coach.

Advice for the Coached Athlete

It sounds simple, but claiming ownership of your own training and progression is both empowering and beneficial. Rather than viewing the coach or program as simply spoon-feeding them with a plan for success, athletes can succeed if they shift their lens to using the coach as a strong resource and technical guide for programming and information. Collaboration is better than a dictatorship, and I urge athletes to be wary of coaches who use terms such as "because I said so" or "because it worked for X." Own your sport, and become an active participant in your own process.

It's important to understand that the coaching process is a journey that can often take a while. I encourage you to commit to the path. Of course it is good to raise questions born out of "healthy skepticism," but a certain level of belief and trust is essential.

As you go on your journey of self-improvement, take note of great athletic success. Whether you get guidance from trusted friends, find a local coach with all the tools, or decide to work with a coach in a predominantly virtual relationship, ensure that you set up your training and performance approach in the way that best suits you. Don't simply assume that the "flavor of the month" is right for you.

Results Are Up to You

"Performance" can mean very different things to different athletes. While I love coaching my elite athletes, I am also inspired by anyone who commits to self-improvement and looks to achieve their own brand of excellence. Within the purplepatch community, we have the well-known list of pros gaining wins and podiums at the top tier of the sport. We also have many others who don't dream of making podiums or taking titles, but they make triathlon a vehicle for their own self-improvement and personal progression. Their journeys are valuable and special in their own right, and every purplepatch athlete, from pro to beginner, can appreciate others' journeys.

Now it is your turn. You can go on and achieve whatever your dreams are in the sport. The education and information are important, and a coach might frame the path and training to guide and help you on your way, but the true results will be owned by you. To commit to your own journey of improvement and your own excellence involves a certain amount of risk and exposure. Many of us—no, all of us—carry at least a small amount of fear of failure and aversion to risk, but those who step forward to begin the journey can never fail. Remember, most of your worries likely won't happen. Take the first step toward your own excellence: Own your journey, and own your results. The rewards are much greater than podiums and titles. Best of luck.

SELF-ASSESSMENT QUESTIONNAIRE WITH ANSWERS

The self-assessment questionnaire appears at the end of Chapter 1. Here are the questions with the coach's answers.

Endurance Training

1. **Is your rating of how your training is going dependent on the number of hours you accumulate in each discipline?** *No. The number of hours or miles you've logged is not a good measure of how successful your training is.*

2. **Do you stick to a regular training template, and are you willing to make changes as you go?** *Yes. It's important to be intentional in your training; however, you also need to be flexible when the feedback you get indicates that something needs to change.*

3. **Do you perform most of your training sessions at a relatively similar intensity?** *No. A progressive plan will include a wide variety of high- and low-intensity sessions. If your plan lacks a variety of easy, moderate, and hard sessions, you need to make a change. If you often end up going hard in easy sessions, you are compromising your training. Keep the hard sessions hard and the easy sessions easy.*

4. **Do you plan for rest and recovery?** *Yes. It's a mistake to assume that there is no need to integrate specific recovery into training.*

5. **Do you follow a classic periodization build of 3 weeks of hard work followed by 1 week of easy work throughout the season?** *No. It's best to take more frequent recovery every 10 to 14 days (or as needed). For most athletes, recovery blocks are 2 to 4 days. Avoid training 3 weeks hard, then taking 1 week of rest. Frequent recovery allows you to get in front of deep fatigue, allowing for higher-quality training sessions on a more consistent basis. The other hallmark of periodization involves focusing a phase of training on one specific purpose (endurance, muscular endurance, speed, etc.). Variation with frequent recovery yields better results.*

6. **Do you place the same emphasis on your swimming training as you do on cycling and running training?** *Yes. Even though swimming is a relatively small part of the full event, that's no reason to cheat your swimming training. Some triathletes haven't seen improvements, so they decide it's not worth the time— not true.*

Nutrition
Daily Nutrition

1. **Do you often limit your caloric intake or try to hit a particular number of calories with your daily diet?** *No. The demands of endurance training require plenty of calories, but this is not a fixed number. That said, it's important to be in control of your intake. If you are overeating or fighting off cravings, that's a warning sign.*

2. **Do you avoid fat in your daily meals and snacks?** *No. Fat plays an important role in the endurance athlete's diet.*

3. **Do you rely on carbohydrates as a main or primary source of calories in most of your meals?** *No. Whole-grain carbohydrates are a good choice, but fruits and vegetables are carbohydrates too—eat plenty of them. A balanced diet should include plenty of protein and fat as well as carbohydrates. You should consider avoiding or limiting starchy carbohydrates in your evening meals.*

4. **Do you frequently skip breakfast or have a hard time consuming calories early in the day?** *No. It is important to consume calories in the morning, as it sets the stage for appropriate eating choices during the rest of the day. Taking in protein when you wake up will lower your stress hormone (cortisol), and absorp-*

tion of carbohydrates is best in the morning. Don't dig yourself a caloric deficit in the morning hours, as it presents a stressful and emotionally challenging approach to food choices later in the day.

5. Do you often go more than 4 hours in the day without consuming any calories? *No. You want to limit caloric excesses to maintain homeostasis (balance) in terms of both deficit and excess. Small, frequent snacks and meals will be easily absorbed and help prevent the stress of "athletic starvation."*

6. Are you able to regulate body composition and energy levels without counting calories or putting yourself on a strict "diet"? *Yes. It's important to learn how to listen to your body as an endurance athlete. Counting calories or maintaining a caloric deficit to lose weight will hurt performance.*

Fueling

1. Do you take in calories for any training session that lasts more than 60 minutes? *Yes. The goal should be to take in 3 to 4 kilocalories (kcal) per kilogram of bodyweight each hour of training. This should be consumed in microdoses every 7 to 20 minutes.*

2. Do you always consume calories within 60 minutes of training? *Yes. You should aim to consume 20 grams of protein within 20 minutes after training, then a balanced and complete meal within the next 60 to 90 minutes.*

3. Do you consume protein within 15 to 20 minutes after most training sessions? *Yes. Even after light sessions, we want to optimize recovery, begin protein synthesis, and lower the cortisol response associated with training. It is a great time to take in protein.*

4. Do you fear taking in calories during or immediately after exercise due to issues with your weight or body composition? *No. Feeding and refueling are essential to limit stress, facilitate recovery, and manage future portion control in daily eating and meals. You will never find balance from limiting calories during and after exercise.*

5. Do you focus on hydrating throughout every session, regardless of temperature or intensity? *Yes. Proper hydration staves off fatigue through preserving* *blood volume as well as helping to prevent core temperature from rising as radically. A rule of thumb is 10 to 15 millileters per kilogram of body weight per hour, taken in consistent and small gulps.*

6. **Following a heavy training session, do you often get strong cravings for carbohydrate later in the day?** *No. If you find yourself craving foods such as chocolate, pizza, pasta, or ice cream, it is a sign that your fueling is insufficient. This will have an effect on recovery and food choices during the rest of the day as well as overall performance.*

7. **Do you retain body fat or struggle to maintain proper body composition despite a heavy training load?** *No. We obviously don't wish to retain too much body fat, and the typical causes are fueling strategies, overstress, or too much training relative to recovery.*

Hydration

1. **Do you consume at least 1 ounce of fluid per pound of body weight on a daily basis?** *Yes. Daily hydration is a key to good performance and balancing energy levels.*

2. **Do you consume any sugar-based beverages (Red Bull, Monster, Coke, etc.) outside exercise?** *No. While there's no need to fret over calories, these beverages deliver no nutritional value. Avoid them.*

3. **During training, do you hydrate with a low-carbohydrate sports drink (under 4 percent solution)?** *Yes. Avoid sports drinks with a high sugar base (Gatorade, Perform, etc.). On the other end of the spectrum, water with electrolytes (Nuun, salt and lime juice, etc.) is not a good match for the demands of training. If you are unsure about the solution of your sports drink, see "Hydration and Thirst" in Chapter 4.*

Functional Strength

1. **Do you follow any strength and conditioning program as part of your triathlon training?** *Yes. If your answer is no, skip to the recovery section of the self-assessment, but note that functional strength should become an area of focus for you. Read Chapter 5 twice. Strength training should happen throughout the season, not just in the off-season or at the first sign of injury.*

2. **Does your functional strength plan evolve in focus throughout the season?** *Yes. As for endurance training, your functional strength plan should be progressive. If it falls off as your racing picks up, you are missing out on performance gains.*

3. **Does your strength training focus on group-based classes such as pilates, yoga, or TRX?** *No. These classes are good for general fitness and health, but they lack the progression and variety that will lead to better performance.*

4. **Do you focus on specific personal weaknesses (mobility, strength, coordination) in your functional strength training?** *Yes. A good program will be tailored to your individual needs. In Chapter 5 you will find a self-assessment to help you shape your program for the best results.*

FUNCTIONAL STRENGTH EXERCISES

What follows is a dive into a selection of functional strength exercises. As I stressed in Chapter 5, you could incorporate any number of exercises into your own individualized program. You'll recall that many of these exercises were used in the snapshots of progressive functional strength sessions for each phase in Chapter 5. Here they are categorized according to their primary *focus:* stability and coordination, mobility, strength, and power. Within each category, the exercises are generally organized to progress from more basic exercises and movements to more complex or difficult exercises; however, what is basic for one athlete might be challenging for another. Use the Functional Strength Self-Assessment (page 99) to select exercises that address your individual strengths and weaknesses. You can find additional exercises at www.purplepatchfitness.com.

Keep in mind that every strength workout should include a dynamic warm-up and some ancillary exercises. Exercises that can be used in this way are called out within their respective categories.

STABILITY & COORDINATION

This is the ability to hold the proper body position (in your sport) either when stationary or, more important, moving. A strong ability to retain central stability is the platform for maintaining form in fatigue as well as maximizing power potential.

BACKWARD LUNGES

FOCUS: lower-body strength & core stability

Improves hip, hamstring, and groin mobility and flexibility; challenges the core and general posture

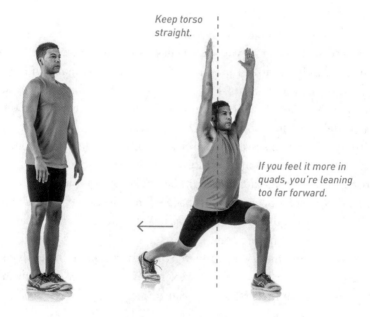

Keep torso straight.

If you feel it more in quads, you're leaning too far forward.

→ Start standing with feet shoulder width apart.

→ Step backward with leg dropping down until knee barely clears the ground. Be sure to control your descent with the stationary leg.

→ Return to standing position and repeat on other side, alternating legs until you finish the set.

Do the lunge on a line or in front of a mirror to make sure you're moving straight back, not out to the side.

HIGH KNEES

FOCUS: hip flexor, core & glute coordination; running posture

Strengthens hip stabilizers, improves hip extension

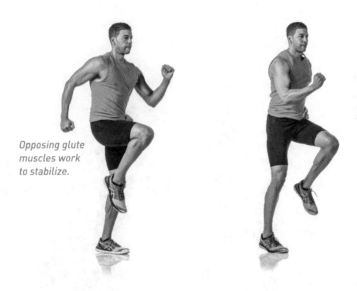

Opposing glute muscles work to stabilize.

→ Stand with arms at sides, head in neutral position.

→ Raise knee to 90 degrees while keeping the other leg straight with knee locked. Use the glute muscles of the standing leg to stabilize.

→ Alternate legs, driving high knee into the ground as opposite leg comes up. This is a fast movement.

If you have trouble balancing, focus on a point ahead of you.

FOCUS: upper- & lower-body coordination

Challenges hip and groin stability, strengthens shoulder rotators

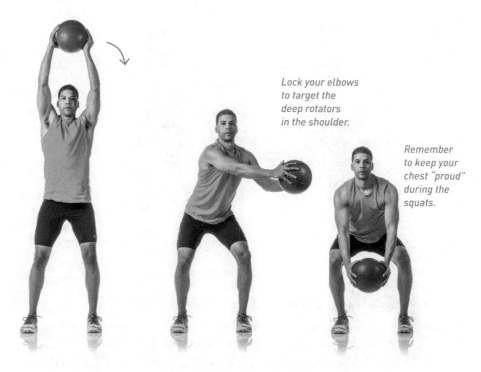

Lock your elbows to target the deep rotators in the shoulder.

Remember to keep your chest "proud" during the squats.

→ Standing with feet shoulder width apart, hold the ball at waist with elbows extended. Raise medicine ball above head.

→ Squat down and rise back up while moving the medicine ball in a clockwise circle.

→ Repeat, moving the medicine ball counterclockwise. Continue alternating direction of movement until you finish the set.

Try circling the ball to hit the overhead position both while you squat to the bottom and while you stand back up.

CARIOCAS

FOCUS: hip mobility & coordination

Opens hips, adductors, and groin

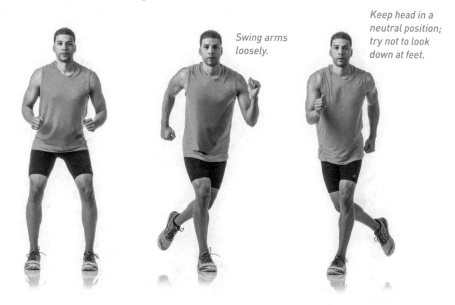

Swing arms loosely.

Keep head in a neutral position; try not to look down at feet.

→ Stand with arms at sides.

→ Jog sideways a few steps in one direction before turning hips to make a "step-over" motion with the trailing leg.

→ Alternate, crossing trailing knee over lead leg.

→ Repeat movement in the opposite direction.

To get the most out of the drill, allow your hips to rotate forward and backward to allow you to move sideways.

CALF RAISES

FOCUS: lower-limb stability & strength

Strengthens calves, feet, and ankles and improves ankle and calf flexibility

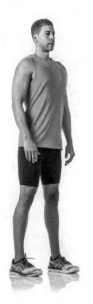
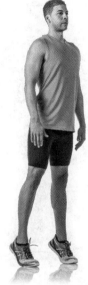

Come over big toe during the raise to maximally train calf.

→ Lock knees and rise up on toes as high as possible.

→ Return to neutral and repeat movement with control until you finish the set.

Go slowly to work all the minor muscles in the ankle. Use a stair or box or step to increase range of motion, dropping heels down and rising up.

SIDE PLANK CLAMS

FOCUS: core stability & hip mobility

Engages the gluteus medius and maximus, problem areas for many
endurance athletes

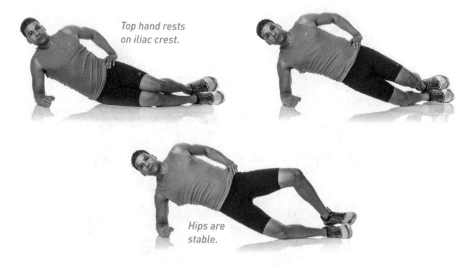

Top hand rests
on iliac crest.

Hips are
stable.

→ Begin in regular side plank position, with knees bent.

→ Lift into side plank, holding position and engaging glutes to gain a
stable platform.

→ Keeping heels together, lift top knee without allowing any rotation in hips.

→ Finish reps, and repeat on other side.

----

*Establish good stability in the side plank position before adding the hip, or "clam," move-
ment. Athletes without the ability to maintain the baseline side plank position will sag at the
hips or rotate the hip when lifting the knee.*

ANTIROTATION PUNCHES

FOCUS: upper-body lateral stability

Forces proper posture and lateral stability, engaging push-and-pull movements common in endurance sports

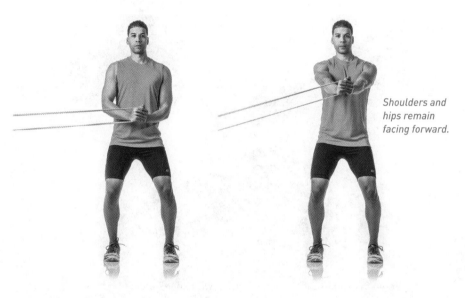

Shoulders and hips remain facing forward.

→ Stand with great posture in neutral position, feet shoulder width apart. Fix band in a lateral position, slightly taut.

→ Maintain posture and stability while pushing out band with both hands as lateral tension increases.

→ Keep shoulders, hips, and knuckles facing forward while driving out slow and steady to full extension.

→ Bring hands back in starting position in a controlled movement.

→ Finish reps, and repeat on other side.

Don't use a band that carries too much gauge and pulls you off from neutral or causes you to lean too much—form over force is the key here.

STANDING CONTRALATERAL PUNCHES

FOCUS: upper-body stability & power

Heightens load of independent stability and coordination, increases lateral stability, optimizes power transfer, and maintains technique when fatigued

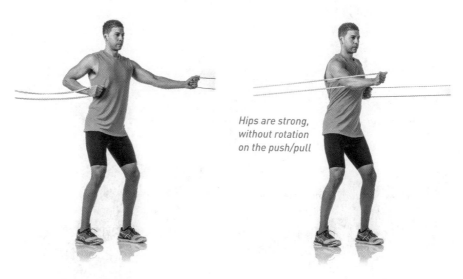

Hips are strong, without rotation on the push/pull

→ Stand with great posture, feet shoulder width apart, with two bands, slightly taut, one anchored in front of you and the other behind you.

→ Maintain posture and stability while pushing band from rear and pulling front band with opposite hand.

→ Keep shoulders, hips, and knuckles facing forward while driving out slowly to full extension and pulling back with opposing hand.

→ Counter resistance and bring hands back into starting position in a controlled movement.

→ Finish reps and repeat, using bands in opposite directions.

This exercise will highlight your weaknesses; a controlled motion is important.

MOBILITY

This concept is different from flexibility, which is the active lengthening of a muscle. Mobility is the natural range of motion around a joint. Retaining or improving joint mobility will enable you to get into the appropriate position to attain proper technique in each discipline, will maximize your optimal movement economy, and will help prevent injury.

SIDE PLANKS

FOCUS: mobility & stability

Simulates a specific stress to help with the manual phase of running

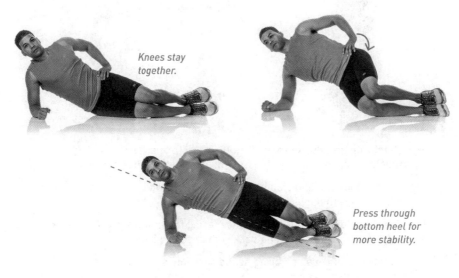

Knees stay together.

Press through bottom heel for more stability.

→ Lie on side with knees bent in front of you. Place elbow directly beneath shoulder and balance on forearm with stacked hips and heels.

→ Slowly raise hips to initiate the exercise and squeeze them forward until shoulders, hips, and knees are in a straight line.

→ Pause, then lower hips back down, controlling the movement.

→ Finish reps, and repeat on other side.

The crooked position of the setup can be tricky and is important to get right. Apply some downward pressure in the supportive forearm to avoid collapsing into the shoulder.

KNEELING HIP EXTENSIONS

FOCUS: lower-body mobility

Activates glute, which plays an important role as a hip extensor during running

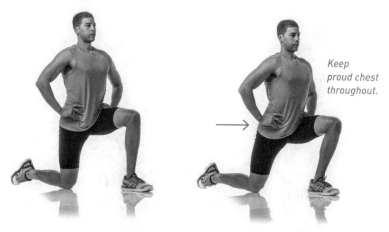

Keep proud chest throughout.

→ Start in split kneeling position with working knee on the ground and a proud chest.

→ Squeeze glute, pushing body forward into lunge.

→ Finish reps, and repeat with opposite knee on the ground.

Your goal is to make the hip angle as wide as possible without falling forward.

WALL ANGELS

FOCUS: upper-body mobility

Improves thoracic mobility and increases range of motion through shoulders

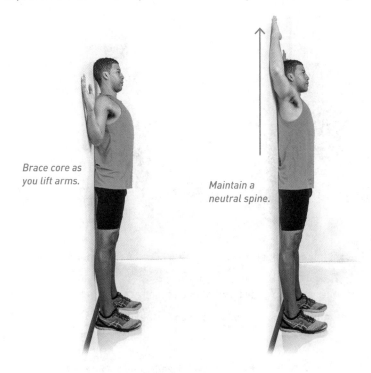

Brace core as you lift arms.

Maintain a neutral spine.

→ Stand with back against the wall, feet hip width apart, elbows bent with arms against the wall.

→ Keeping elbows and hands against the wall, slowly lift arms until fingertips touch overhead.

→ Stay tall, then slowly lower arms to sides, keeping elbows bent.

Try not to peel away from the wall or arch your back. Think about squeezing your shoulder blades as you lower your arms.

FACE-THE-WALL SQUATS

FOCUS: lower-body mobility

Teaches how to use glutes throughout the squat so as not to overrely on the quads

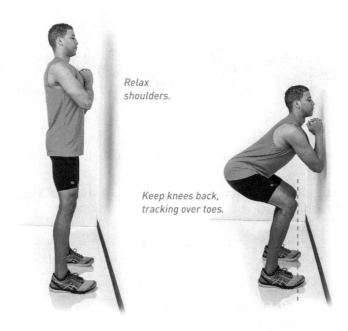

Relax shoulders.

Keep knees back, tracking over toes.

→ Face the wall, standing about elbow's length away. Legs are shoulder width apart, and toes point out slightly.

→ Look straight ahead as you push hips back and lower body into squat without touching the wall.

→ Pause, then slowly rise back up to the starting position.

Keep the weight off your toes so you don't roll forward. If your knees touch the wall, you won't be able to squat down.

RIB ROLLS

FOCUS: upper-body mobility

Improves rotation in anticipation of body rotation during swim and arm swing on run

Feel core muscles engage.

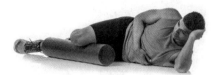 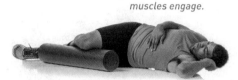

→ Lie on side. Bend elbow to support head on hand. Elbow should point forward.

→ Rest upper arm on side, with hand resting on lower ribs. Bend upper knee and place it on a foam roller or medicine ball positioned slightly in front of you.

→ Lower upper shoulder blade to the floor behind you. Supporting elbow will lift as shoulder drops, and lower rib cage also will twist and rotate up.

→ Lift shoulder to roll back to the start position.

→ Finish reps, and repeat on other side.

Really try to glue your shoulder blade to your ribs to get the full benefit of the rotation. It is easy to roll your shoulders back toward the floor, but the aim is to rotate the entire rib cage. It takes focus and practice. Note that you can likely rotate much farther one way than the other!

QUADRUPED HIP FLEXIONS/EXTENSIONS

FOCUS: mobility & stability

Improves postural fitness on the bike and lateral stability on the run

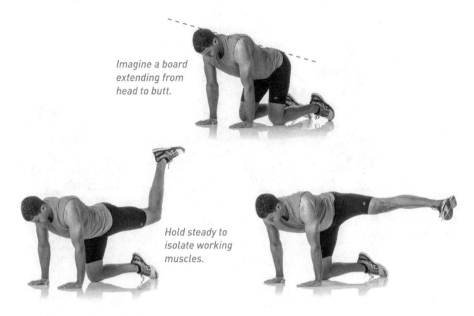

Imagine a board extending from head to butt.

Hold steady to isolate working muscles.

→ Begin in a tabletop position, with knees aligned under hips and hands shoulder width apart. This exercise is two distinct movements:

Hip Flexion: Drive leg back until quad is parallel to the floor. Finish reps, and repeat on other side.

Hip Extension: Swing leg out laterally until knee is aligned with hip. Finish reps, and repeat on other side.

Avoid rushing these movements. Some quality motion in the hip is better than getting extra motion by substituting the back as the prime mover.

GOBLET RIDE-DOWNS WITH REACH

FOCUS: lower- & upper-body mobility

Improves hip mobility, which is a problem for a lot of endurance athletes

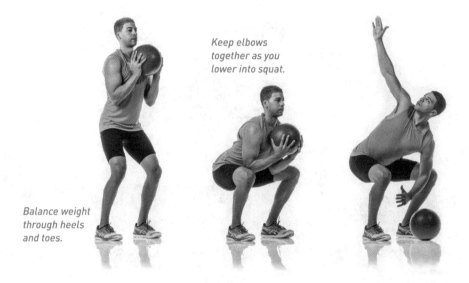

Keep elbows together as you lower into squat.

Balance weight through heels and toes.

→ Stand with elbows forward and forearms pressed together. Palms will be open, facing straight up, to hold medicine ball (as if it were a goblet).

→ Carry ball down into a squat, staying stable and controlled throughout the movement.

→ At bottom of squat, release ball. Rotate torso and reach upward with one arm.

→ Pick up ball, and return to start position. Repeat, alternating reach, until set is complete.

Y'S, T'S, W'S

FOCUS: upper-body mobility & stability

A great range-of-motion exercise designed to keep shoulders and thoracic spine mobile and strong

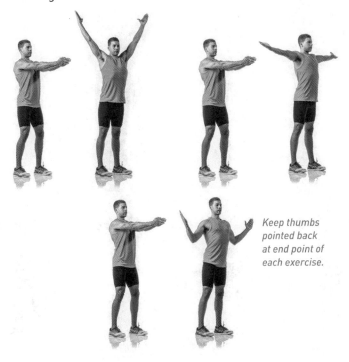

Keep thumbs pointed back at end point of each exercise.

→ Standing tall with a proud chest, reach straight in front of you with palms facing each other.

→ Staying tall, bring both arms back up over shoulders to make a "Y" between body and arms.

→ Return to start position.

→ Next, keeping arms at shoulder height; bring arms back with elbows straight to the side, making the "T."

→ Return to start position.

→ Finally, let elbows bend slightly while bringing arms back slightly below chest height, making a "W."

→ Repeat sequence until set is complete.

Try not to let your chest and head drift forward as you bring arms back.

Y'S, T'S, W'S WITH BANDS

FOCUS: upper-body mobility & stability

A great range-of-motion exercise designed to keep shoulders and thoracic spine mobile and strong

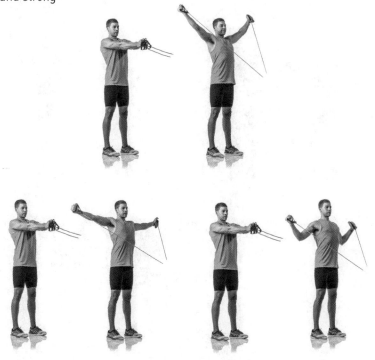

→ Anchor resistance tubing in front of you at about chest height. Standing tall with proud chest, reach straight in front of you with palms facing each other.

→ Staying tall, pull both arms back up over shoulders to make a "Y" between body and arms.

→ Return to start position.

→ Next, keeping arms at shoulder height; pull arms back with elbows straight to the side, making the "T."

→ Return to start position.

→ Finally, let elbows bend slightly while pulling arms back slightly below chest height, making a "W."

→ Repeat sequence until set is complete.

Try not to let your chest and head drift forward as you bring arms back.

STRENGTH

Strength alone won't improve endurance performance, but increasing the contractile ability of the muscle and increasing the numbers of muscle fibers in the usable mix will improve your potential for power production in all three sports as well as your resistance to fatigue. Put simply, strength is the extent to which muscles can exert force by contracting against load, or resistance.

ELBOW-TO-KNEE LUNGES

FOCUS: lower-body strength & balance

Improves hip, hamstring, and groin mobility and flexibility; challenges balance

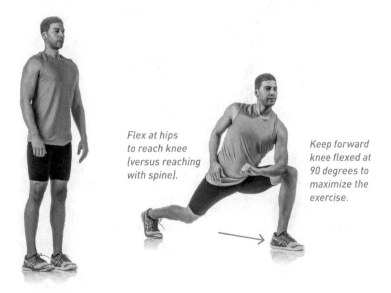

Flex at hips to reach knee (versus reaching with spine).

Keep forward knee flexed at 90 degrees to maximize the exercise.

→ Start in normal standing position.

→ Lunge forward with one leg, keeping knee over big toe. Touch elbow to inside of forward knee.

→ Return to standing position.

→ Repeat on other side, alternating until set is complete.

If you find yourself losing your balance, you might be lunging too far forward.

SINGLE-LEG ROMANIAN DEADLIFTS

FOCUS: lower-body strength & core stability

Improves stability and power on the bike and run

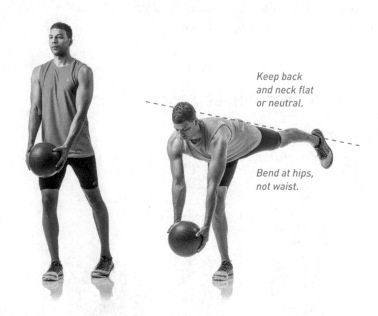

Keep back
and neck flat
or neutral.

Bend at hips,
not waist.

→ Standing on one leg, hold weight in both hands or in opposite hand.

→ Bend forward at hip, keeping knee slightly bent and back flat.

→ Lower weight to just above floor.

→ Squeeze glute muscle to return to start position.

→ Finish reps, and repeat on other side.

Control the motion as much as possible—avoid the temptation to teeter back and forth.

MEDICINE-BALL SQUATS

FOCUS: lower-body strength

Develops strength and stability in major muscles used in riding and running

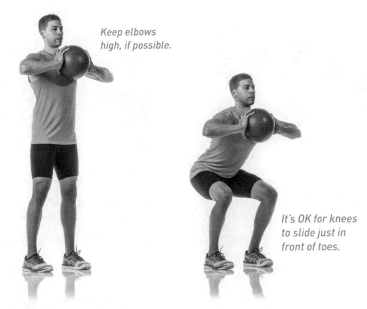

Keep elbows high, if possible.

It's OK for knees to slide just in front of toes.

→ Standing with feet shoulder width apart, hold a medicine ball at chest height.

→ Push hips back, keep chest proud, and "sit back" as if into a chair.

→ Continue descending until you reach a 90-degree position at the shin and thigh.

→ Reverse motion to return to start position.

Try "ripping the floor apart" by attempting to turn your feet out on the way back up to feel more gluteal activation.

PUSH-UPS, WIDE

FOCUS: general strength & core stability

Stabilizes and strengthens shoulder muscles used in swimming and enhances core stability

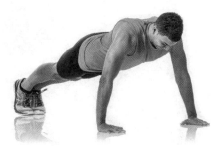

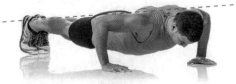

Don't let body sag; maintain good posture.

→ Place hands in a slightly wider grip than a traditional push-up, just outside shoulders. Keep body straight and taut throughout the exercise.

→ Pull body down into the floor, maintaining a tight position, then drive back up to the starting position.

Maintain broadness through your neck and shoulders to hold the "T" position as you lower to the floor.

FRONT LUNGES

FOCUS: lower-body strength

A popular exercise in functional strength for endurance athletes; goal is perfect symmetry

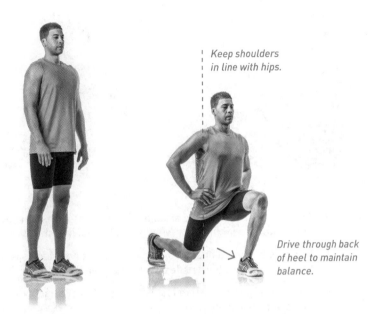

Keep shoulders in line with hips.

Drive through back of heel to maintain balance.

→ Stand with feet shoulder width apart and hands on hips. Upper body is upright and proud.

→ In one fluid movement, lift one knee and take a big step forward, placing foot in front of body. Drop hips forward and down into the lunge.

→ Pause, keeping upper leg parallel to the floor; then, in another fluid movement, push off front foot back to starting position.

→ Repeat, alternating legs, until set is complete.

To synchronize more movement in the lunge, alternate opposite arm to leg: for example, as right leg lunges forward, left arm comes forward and right arm goes back. This is similar to a running motion.

SEATED ROWS

FOCUS: secondary upper-body strength

Helps with general upper-body strength and the pull components of swimming

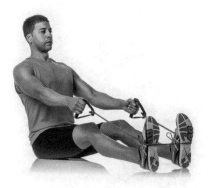
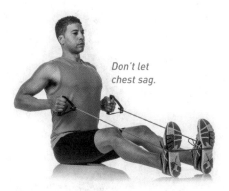

Don't let chest sag.

→ Anchor a resistance band around a fixed object in front of you, or your feet, and sit upright on the floor with legs extended in front.

→ Begin with a proud chest, holding the band in both hands with some tension. Start pulling shoulder blades back, and then draw elbows back.

→ Pull bands until hands are just below chest. Move back to starting position in a controlled manner.

If you want to make it harder, choke up on the resistance band to increase tension.

FRONT SQUATS

FOCUS: lower-body strength & core stability

Improves basic strength and mobility and strengthens core and lower back

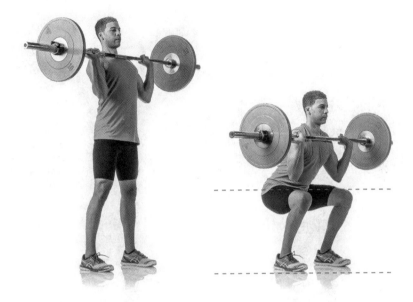

→ Stand with a proud chest. Support bar across chest and shoulders with wrists back and palms up.

→ Start front squat by unseating hips. Squat down until quads are parallel with the floor. Pause, then press up until back at starting position.

Incorporate the whole body, not just your quads and legs, throughout the exercise. If you are new to Olympic lifts, hold the bar with arms crossed—this is the safest position (see below).

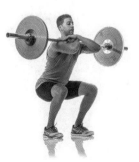

STANDING SHOULDER PRESSES

FOCUS: upper-body strength & core

Strengthens torso; teaches sequencing of legs, core, and upper body

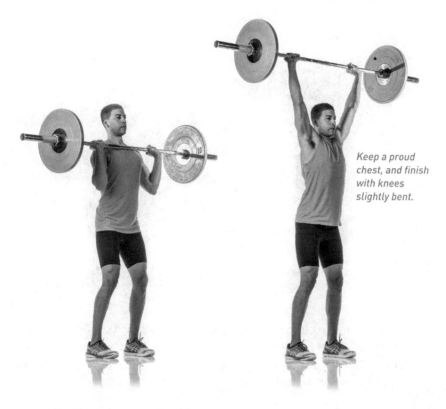

Keep a proud chest, and finish with knees slightly bent.

→ Position bar across shoulders and chest with wrists back and palms up.

→ Drop hips slightly, then push ground away, driving bar off shoulders.

→ As legs fully extend, push bar all the way up, causing arms to lock.

→ Lower bar to starting position in a controlled manner.

You may rise up onto your toes on the drive phase, but try not to leave the ground; the bulk of the force is produced by the legs creating momentum for the bar. To reduce load, use dumbbells.

HIGH STEP-UPS WITH WEIGHT

FOCUS: lower-body strength & core

Single-leg drill great for developing stability, strength, and balance with minimal load

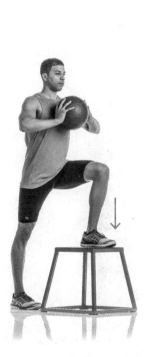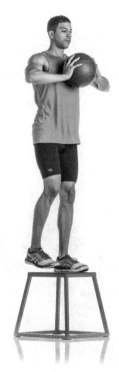

→ Place one foot on a box/step at approximately knee height.

→ Putting weight through lead leg as much as possible, push down and step all the way up onto the box.

→ Pause, then reverse the motion to lower back down to the starting position.

→ Repeat with opposite leg, alternating legs until set is complete.

There are many variations to this exercise, and we've chosen to show an advanced version. Most people should start with a platform below knee height.

POWER

Power has something to do with strength, but only when we add another element: speed. Power is the ability to exert high force through a short period of time. Moving load *fast* is the recipe for improving power potential.

SINGLE-LEG BOUNDS DYNAMIC WARM-UP

FOCUS: Explosive power & speed building

Improves speed and lower-limb strength

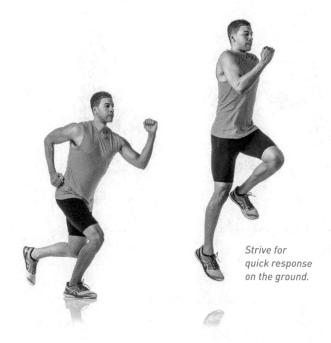

Strive for quick response on the ground.

→ Start in standing position with feet shoulder width apart.

→ Take a few steps to get moving, then jump one-legged from one foot to the other.

As you get more proficient, you can jump farther and higher. Start with a distance and height that are manageable.

PROPULSIONS ABOVE KNEE

FOCUS: dynamic technique & mechanics

Begins teaching the body to use the strength and power hidden in muscles

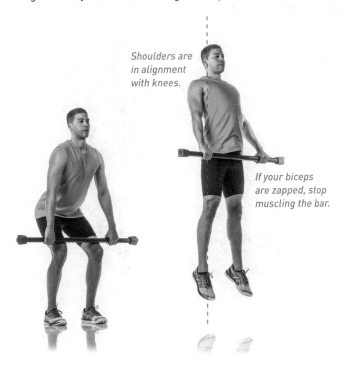

Shoulders are in alignment with knees.

If your biceps are zapped, stop muscling the bar.

→ Stand with a proud chest and knees bent slightly to align over toes. Turn toes slightly outward.

→ Position bar to hang just above knees. Increase bend in knees, then push the floor away and blast off.

→ Land with knees slightly bent and aligned over toes.

Remember, this is a complete-body exercise. The goal is to synchronize legs, hips, core, and shoulders to create a single powerful movement by recruiting muscle that's already there.

PROPULSIONS MIDSHIN

FOCUS: dynamic technique & mechanics

Coordinates legs, hips, core, and shoulders to produce one movement with bar dropped lower to produce more force

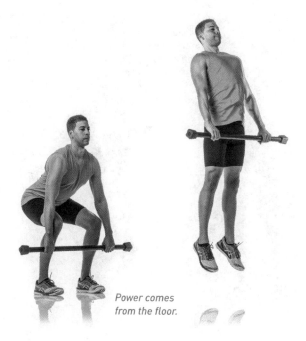

Power comes
from the floor.

→ Stand with proud chest and knees bent slightly to align over toes.

→ Increase bend in knees, then push the floor away and blast off.

→ Land with knees slightly bent and aligned over toes.

If your biceps are zapped, you were muscling the bar too much.

TUCK JUMPS WITH ARMS

FOCUS: power development

Develops explosive power and synchronization in movement associated with riding and running

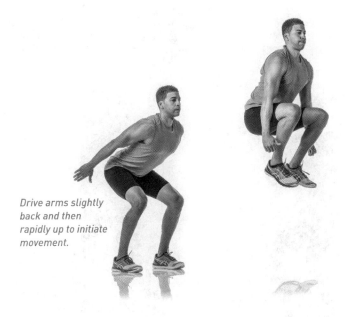

Drive arms slightly back and then rapidly up to initiate movement.

→ Stand with feet shoulder width apart, elbows slightly bent, and hands at hip height.

→ Dip to a one-quarter squat, then immediately blast off, jumping as high as possible.

→ As you reach maximum height, pull knees to chest as high as possible.

→ Land on both feet with a slight knee and ankle bend, ready to take off again.

Many variations are available; try with and without large contributions from the arms.

STANDING PUSH JERKS

FOCUS: power development

Improves total-body explosive power and synchronization

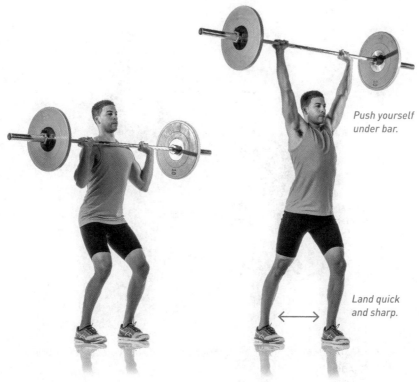

Push yourself under bar.

Land quick and sharp.

→   Stand with feet hip width apart.

→   Place barbell on shoulders, keeping chest proud and knees slightly bent.

→   Drop hips slightly, then push the ground away, driving bar off shoulders.

→   As legs extend, forcefully lock arms while landing in split stance with one knee slightly forward and hip slightly bent.

Depending on your level or access to proper strength equipment, you may use dumbbells or a medicine ball instead of a bar.

HANG CLEAN HIGH PULLS

FOCUS: power development & coordination

Forces neuromuscular synchronization with power development that transfers to swim, bike, and run

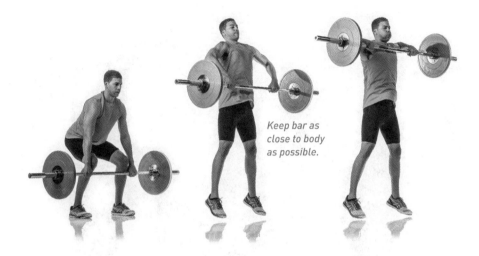

Keep bar as close to body as possible.

→ Start with feet just outside shoulder width and bar resting at hips. To position feet, imagine you are about to jump vertically as high as possible.

→ Slide bar down thighs, pushing hips back to rest just below the kneecaps (same position as Propulsions Midshin).

→ Keeping hips high and weight on heels, start the bar moving by extending hips.

→ As bar moves, perform a jump by rapidly extending ankles, knees, and hips.

→ Using momentum from the jump, shrug shoulders straight up, keeping elbows high.

→ Lower bar back to start position in a controlled manner.

Practice slowly to feel the momentum on the bar before speeding up. Form and technique are critical to force the chain of recruited muscles to be in harmony and to maximize full power potential.

Most athletes will not get to this exercise; we show it for those with more athletic or lifting background. Remember, for our purposes lighter is often better.

FRONT SQUAT TO PUSH PRESSES

FOCUS: power development & strength

Improves hip stability, muscular strength, and power, which transfer to actions in both riding and running

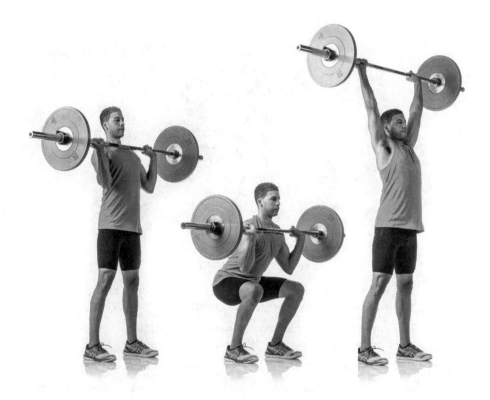

→ Begin with feet shoulder width apart and supple knees. Place bar on upper chest and across shoulders, with wrists back and palms up.

→ Drop into a squat position with controlled movements, pressing weight into heels.

→ Drive out of squat position, pressing bar high overhead in one explosive movement. Finish at full extension through arms.

→ Lower bar back to start position in a controlled movement.

Depending on your level or access to proper strength equipment, you may use dumbbells or a medicine ball instead of a bar.

SCOOP TOSSES

FOCUS: power

Develops power and coordination

Be careful not to twist through spine.

→ Stand with feet just wider than shoulder width.

→ Bend at hips and hold ball close to outside foot.

→ Scoop ball up and over opposite shoulder as far as possible.

→ Finish reps, and repeat on opposite side.

Done well, this exercise might cause you to leave the ground on the toss.

STEP-UPS FAST

FOCUS: lower-body power

Improves synchronization of movement and power development in running

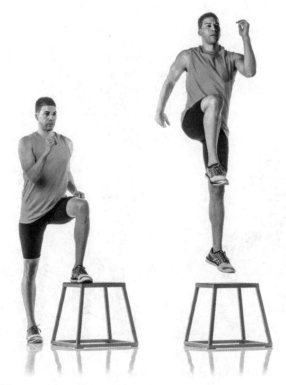

→   Place one foot on top of box.

→   Push off with both legs, blasting high above the box.

→   Switch legs in air, landing with opposite leg on the box and other foot on the ground.

→   Spend as little time on the ground as possible before blasting off again.

Add weight and load as you progress.

TRAINING TEMPLATES

It's easier to keep a clear vision of the training week if you know what workouts are the foundational sessions—the workouts not to be missed. While the entire fabric of your training plan is important, outlining the key sessions and the supporting sessions of each week helps to formulate a decision-making process, facilitates your understanding when you need to be ready to go to work and when to focus on recovery and form, and gives you the ability to trim and adjust if life events get in the way.

In Chapter 10 I structured the sample training blocks in a typical weekly design, but there is always more than one way to achieve an effective training plan. We all have busy lives, with different opportunities to train and recover. The weekly templates that follow are some of the other options that I provide to my athletes. The typical design fits the athlete focused on training, but by moving around the key sessions, we can meet the demands of different lifestyles. You might not find the holy grail for your training week, but you can use these templates as a reference to help you come up with a template of your own.

Remember that the key sessions (highlighted in the templates) are the bedrock of any training week. If you need to reduce your training week, always dial back or remove the supporting sessions first, as they are intended for recovery, general endurance, or setting up the key sessions. Even when you are fatigued or busy, you can still retain the focus and specificity of a training week.

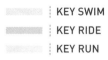

KEY SWIM

KEY RIDE

KEY RUN

THE SAN FRANCISCO ┆ Master Template

	WORKOUT 1	WORKOUT 2
M	Key RIDE	Functional Strength + Optional RUN
T	Key SWIM	Optional RUN
W	Key RIDE	Optional RUN Off the Bike
T	Optional SWIM	Key RUN
F	Key SWIM	Optional RIDE
S	RIDE (recommended)	—
S	Optional SWIM	Key RUN

This template mimics the key sessions and framework of the San Francisco crew.

THE 3-2 PATTERN

	WORKOUT 1	WORKOUT 2
M	Functional Strength + Optional RUN OR REST	—
T	Key SWIM	Key RIDE
W	Key RUN	Optional SWIM
T	Key RIDE	Optional Run Off the Bike
F	Optional RIDE	Functional Strength + Optional RUN
S	RIDE (recommended) Optional Run Off the Bike	P.M. OFF OR Optional SWIM
S	Key SWIM	Key RUN

This template delivers a more classical purplepatch approach, with 3 days in a row of load, 1 day lighter, then 2 days in a row of load, 1 day lighter. It is a good option for many athletes.

OPTION 3

THE WEEKENDER PATTERN

	WORKOUT 1	WORKOUT 2
M	**Functional Strength + Optional SWIM** OR **REST**	—
T	**Key SWIM**	—
W	**Key RUN**	—
T	**Key RIDE** **RUN Off the Bike**	—
F	**Key SWIM**	—
S	**RIDE** (recommended) **RUN Off the Bike**	**Functional Strength + Optional RUN** OR **Optional SWIM**
S	**Key RIDE**	**Key RUN**

This template is for athletes who can do only one session per day on weekdays and plan to load a little more training into their weekends.

OPTION 4

THE SLEEPY SUNDAY PATTERN

	WORKOUT 1	WORKOUT 2
M	**Key RIDE** **RUN Off the Bike**	—
T	**Key SWIM**	**Key RUN**
W	**Key RIDE**	**Functional Strength + Optional Swim**
T	**Key SWIM**	**Key RUN**
F	**Functional Strength + Optional SWIM** OR **Optional RIDE**	—
S	**RIDE** (recommended) **RUN Off the Bike**	—
S	**Functional Strength + Optional SWIM** OR **Optional RIDE** OR **REST**	*This day is interchangeable with Saturday.*

This template is for athletes who are family- or social-focused and wish to make at least one weekend day a rest day (day off or minimal training).

ACKNOWLEDGMENTS

There is great strength to be had in surrounding oneself with smart, passionate people, especially when they are masters of their own craft. I am very lucky to have people both inside and outside triathlon who are willing to provide me with guidance, thoughts, and education in their areas of expertise. They are willing to challenge me and my ideas, and these challenges have allowed me to grow as a person and a coach.

Unfortunately, there is not space in the book to highlight each and every supporter, adviser, or resource who has helped me throughout my coaching career and the writing of this book, but I would like to acknowledge a few individuals who have shaped my coaching methodology and helped with this process.

The Heavy Lifters

JOHN BALL is an invaluable resource to me as a coach and an inspiration on the topic of functional strength as well as injury prevention and treatment. John is one of the smart ones, and his dedication to his craft and helping athletes, his contribution to the purplepatch program over the past several years, and his assistance with the functional strength chapter in this book cannot be overstated.

PAUL BUICK has become an integral part of the purplepatch coaching family in recent years. A true craftsman of the bicycle, Paul brings expertise on riding position and posture, handling skills, and how to excel on the bike. Beyond all this, Paul has a wonderful coaching eye for the individual athlete. His knowledge and understanding of how to approach cycling in triathlon exceed those of anyone else I have encountered in the sport. He is a hidden gem, and I believe he has the knowledge and expertise to change the way triathlon riding is approached.

GERRY RODRIGUES is my "partner in crime" when it comes to coaching. He has been a mentor, adviser, and guide in coaching open-water swimming and much more. I believe every coach needs mentors and supporters, and Gerry is one of my most trusted resources. I was lucky enough to swim under Gerry's coaching during my pro career, and in the years since then we have developed a strong friendship.

The Supporting Cast

I believe in looking beyond the sport for inspiration and guidance in training, coaching, mind-set, and athlete management. I am lucky to receive guidance, discussions, and insight from business leaders, coaches, and athletes in other sports. Many have been instrumental in helping me with the lessons of coaching and planning, and I have been lucky to adapt and apply these lessons to our sport. Stacy Sims is my best resource on fueling, nutrition, hydration, and all things physiology (www.osmonutrition.com). Matthew Weatherly-White is a smart chap in all things training and recovery and a heck of an athlete himself (www.restwise.com). I consider Garret Rock one of the good guys, a great resource for the health of my athletes. Tim O'Neill is a smart guy in functional movement and strength (www.ceaqc.com).

A massive thank-you to my passionate and hardworking team at purplepatch as well as the entire purplepatch family of athletes and supporters. You know who you are, and your help and passion are noted and appreciated.

A Final Thank-You

Where would I be without the support of the many people who have supported me personally on this journey so far? My wife, Kelli, who supports, pushes, and loves me through it all, and Baxter, my son, who wonders why Daddy likes whistles and stopwatches. My brothers, Martin and Peter, who provided life education through constant sporting (and sometimes physical) beatings when I was a youngster and always pushed me toward excellence and a big life. My mum, Mary, for being Mum and for taking me swimming too much and too often as a little boy, enough to make me sweat the smell of chlorine. Who knew where all this would end? My friends Peter and Carmel, who spend too many days and nights listening. And all the other people who add passion and fun to my life.

This book is dedicated to my dad, Norman Dixon. He loved to teach and loved to help; he was a kind and gentle man. I will never forget all he did, including so much work to help me receive a sports scholarship to swim at a university in the United States and get this journey started. I wouldn't have started my journey without his help. He was in the process of writing a book on teaching swimming when he passed away, and his book was never finished. I never dreamed that I would now be finishing a book on coaching in endurance sports, and I cannot imagine finishing this without a nod of love and gratitude to him.

INDEX

best/maximal, 209; maximal, 137, 205; sustainable, 133–134, 181, 285

Elbow-to-knee lunges, described, 317

Electrolytes, 72, 74, 286

Emotions, 36, 38, 115, 127, 136, 181, 236; focusing, 144, 224

Endurance, 1, 9, 10, 17, 39, 62, 77, 87, 112, 202, 204, 207, 210, 232, 241, 242, 272, 273, 280; cardiovascular, 131, 201; equipment-strip, 129–132; focus on, 173, 230; foundation of, 133, 240, 288; improving, 129, 131, 173, 197, 205, 206, 230, 231; interval, 132–133; lower-intensity, 176, 238, 248; lower-stress, 175, 201; maintaining, 55, 205, 208;   medium, 33; muscular, 111, 118, 122–123, 131, 133, 173, 204, 206, 229, 248; nutrition and, 61; performance and, 67; short-rep, 130–131; strength and, 8, 231

Endurance training, 1–5, 7, 9, 10, 25, 78, 79, 231, 293, 297; blood and, 73; goals for, 30–33; pre-season, 84, 85; questions about, 12; strength training and, 87; stress and, 17; tension-variance, 175

Energy, 38, 63, 67, 71, 72, 73, 127, 269, 279; cost, 115, 140, 143; emotional, 115, 136, 181, 189; gaining, 41, 158, 266; loss of, 286; maintaining, 32, 75, 76, 143; saving, 116, 126, 171

English, Clif, 291

Entry, 119 (fig.)

Equipment, 126, 145, 148, 150, 267–268, 277, 286

Execution, 189, 240, 268, 277, 278, 279

Exercise, 299; improving, 11; low-intensity, 243; maintaining, 244; warm-up, 89

Experience, 88–89, 135, 220

F

Face-the-wall squats, 91 (fig.), 96, 103 (fig.); described, 311

Fat, 62, 69, 71, 249, 294; consuming, 75; fueling with, 9, 63; storing, 10, 57, 63, 65

Fatigue, 3, 25, 37, 47, 48, 49, 73, 79, 86, 189, 190, 193, 197, 202, 220, 231, 232, 235, 244, 247, 251, 265, 268, 270, 271, 279, 280, 290; accumulated, 5, 26, 28, 29 (table), 31, 38, 43, 66, 186, 230, 236, 241; excessive, 21, 27, 51, 66, 273; freedom from, 198; impact of, 196; levels of, 18; massive, 198, 236,

269; readiness and, 39; recovering from, 222; residual, 28, 200, 201, 271; risk of, 228; running and, 186, 200, 201; soreness and, 84; training and, 9, 70

Feedback, 1, 38, 115–116, 160, 216, 280, 289, 293

Filliol, Joel, 291

Fitness, 18, 32, 131, 178, 191, 199, 202, 215, 221, 266, 269, 287, 288; aerobic, 9, 229; benchmarks for, 216; cardiovascular, 170; decline in, 55, 271; foundation of, 133, 171, 174, 220, 229; improving, 10, 42, 44, 115, 127, 136, 173, 176, 232, 233, 270; level of, 28, 197, 229; performance and, 67, 118, 265; postural, 145, 152, 153–154 (fig.), 155, 156, 164, 182; swimming and, 115, 129

Fluids, 69, 71, 74, 244

Focus, 6, 111–112, 120, 144, 158, 178, 207, 223, 229, 275, 280; evolving, 39, 188; narrowing, 278–279

Food, 58, 75; choosing, 74, 295, 296; emotional attachment to, 75; high-quality, 7, 62, 69

Force production, 81, 85, 98, 150, 156

Form, 144, 195, 198, 202, 207, 230, 278; executing, 204; force and, 98; improving, 187, 188, 203, 208, 229; load and, 82; maintaining, 201, 209

Forward lean, exaggerating, 192

Forward swing, minimizing, 193

Foundation, 96, 197, 201, 240

Foundational strength, 82, 83–84, 96, 187

Frequency, 186, 198, 201, 202

Front lunges, 91 (fig.); described, 321

Front squat to push presses, 94 (fig.); described, 332

Front squats, 92, 92 (fig.), 96; described, 323

Fueling, 2, 4, 6, 23, 31, 40, 48, 62, 63, 189, 209, 216, 235, 266, 276, 277, 278, 286; benefits of, 66–68; focus on, 275; high-quality, 250; inadequate, 8, 10, 30, 296; nutrition and, 64, 66, 68–72; post-training, 58, 70, 71; postexercise, 204, 250; priority for, 271; proper, 42, 45, 58, 61, 74; questions about, 13; strategies for, 72, 296; training, 63, 69–70, 70 (table); window, 67, 69, 74; windy conditions and, 164

Functional strength, 4, 6, 8, 10, 11, 35, 82–86, 89, 187, 198, 202, 296–297; assessing, 83, 95, 99, 299; exercises for, 299; improving, 77; programs for, 78, 82, 97; questions

of, 5, 21, 23, 30, 41, 57, 247; adaptation
and, 17, 19–27; cardiovascular, 21, 141,
171; handling, 38, 222; hormonal, 21,
23, 42, 219, 269; increasing, 10, 12,
20; life, 21, 24 (fig.), 26, 27, 30, 219,
220, 222; metabolic, 42, 67, 69, 221;
musculoskeletal, 21, 197; nontraining,
20, 21, 28; optimizing, 19–27; physical,
42, 52; physiological, 244; postural, 142,
159; quantifying, 21–23; recovery and,
20; reducing, 67, 133, 171, 198, 201;
responding to, 22, 24, 25, 38, 67, 70, 222;
training, 19, 20, 23, 27–28, 30, 31, 171,
175, 219, 220, 222, 235, 244
Stressors, 20, 23, 25; balancing, 171;
minimizing, 30
Stretching, 46–47, 105
Stroke, 118, 282; breathing and, 122, 123–124;
distance and, 111, 112, 121; freestyle, 111;
long, 112; pull phase of, 118; recovery
phase of, 117, 124; sighting and, 125;
turnover of, 112
Stroke rate, 113, 122; elevated, 122;
eliminating, 111; higher, 121; slower, 122
Structure, 5, 128, 248
Success, 26, 30, 39, 58, 70, 170, 224, 270, 278,
286, 290; achieving, 40, 218; projected, 32;
training and, 21; traits of, 223
Supplementation, 54, 275
Sutton, Brett, 291
Swimmers: middle- to lower-level, 283; upper-
to middle-pack, 282
Swimmer's shoulder, 100
Swimming, 44, 101, 171, 182, 185, 190, 228,
249, 281–282; competitive, 113, 116,
121; fears/anxiety about, 109, 135; fitness
and, 115, 129; focus on, 110, 117, 127,
129; front-quadrant, 112; importance of,
111, 114–115; improving, 109, 113, 114,
115–117, 127, 131, 215, 217; load in, 127,
131, 205, 215; myths of, 111–114; open-
water, 112–113, 114, 116, 117, 120, 122,
123–126, 129, 135, 136; pacing, 282–283;
performance, 126, 127, 217, 248–249; post-
season, 129; race-simulation, 136–137;
technical foundations for, 117, 122;
technique for, 114, 119 (fig.), 123; training
for, 114, 115, 117, 122, 124, 127, 133,
135, 238, 294; triathlon, 109, 110, 111,
114–115, 120, 127–138
Swing action, 193
Synchronization, 80, 82, 84–85, 96 (fig.)

ABOUT THE CONTRIBUTORS

Over the years, I've sought out partnerships that reinforce the purplepatch pillars of performance and deliver more depth and expertise to my athletes. These individuals are among the best in their respective industries, and each of them has made a significant contribution to this book.

DR. JOHN BALL is a second-generation chiropractor who hails from the birthplace of the chiropractic profession, Davenport, Iowa. John attended Arizona State University, where he was a member of the track and cross-country teams, before returning to Iowa to pursue his chiropractic degree at Palmer College. John has extensive postgraduate training in rehabilitation, soft-tissue techniques, and performance training. He holds credentials as an American Chiropractic Board of Sports Physicians Certified Chiropractic Sports Physician (CCSP) and a National Strength and Conditioning Association Certified Strength and Conditioning Specialist (CSCS). John consults with athletes from the NFL and MLB as well as numerous USA track and field athletes. Find out more at www.getmaxmobility.com.

PAUL BUICK is a leading resource in cycling position and posture and technical development. He has a unique ability to go beyond the simple fit and true expertise in assisting athletes in their interactions with the bicycle and in maximizing riding ability. He has extensive experience as a mechanic, technician, and coach for national and professional cycling teams; he has also assisted New Zealand's national triathlon team with riding skills and technical development. He now manages all riding skills, technical development, and fit and posture for most purplepatch professional athletes, and he is assistant coach to Matt Dixon at purplepatch fitness (www.purplepatchfitness.com).

GERRY RODRIGUES is founder and head coach of Tower 26, an open-water swimming program based in Santa Monica, California. A leading technician and strategist of the sport of triathlon and open-water swimming, Gerry has coached some of the world's leading open-water swimmers, Olympic swimmers, and triathletes and Ironman world champions. Find out more at www.tower26.com.

ABOUT THE AUTHOR

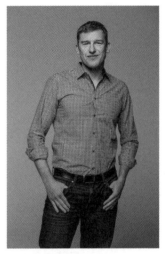

MATT DIXON is an exercise physiologist and an elite coach. He is founder and president of purplepatch fitness, a fitness and coaching company that caters to triathletes and endurance enthusiasts of all levels, from world champions to novices. His clients include leading professional triathletes and endurance athletes, executives of global companies, serious amateur triathletes, and fitness aficionados looking to improve their life and performance. Every purplepatch athlete shares the same goal: a desire for improved performance.

Over the past few years, purplepatch athletes have laid claim to over 150 professional Ironman- and half-Ironman-distance championships and podium finishes, 50 of which have been wins. The winning formula is rooted in Matt Dixon's pillars of performance. When endurance, strength, nutrition, and recovery are adequately and equally developed, athletes enter into a "purple patch" in which top performances become a reality. Matt has developed numerous athletes from the amateur ranks to have highly successful professional careers. He has also helped more than 100 athletes qualify for and compete in the Hawaii Ironman World Championship.

Matt's coaching career is steeped in his own experience, first as an elite swimmer and then as a professional triathlete. He was a two-time Olympic trials finalist for Great Britain and an NCAA Division I swimmer. His triathlon career spanned multiple seasons; he competed as a pro at the Hawaii Ironman and won Vineman 70.3.

Starting out as a coach in a national champion swimming program, Matt went on to become an NCAA Division 1 collegiate swimming coach while completing his master's degree in clinical and exercise physiology. He ultimately landed in triathlon and has been coaching triathletes for over 10 years.

Matt is a regular columnist and/or contributor to *Triathlete* magazine, *Triathlete Europe*, and *Lava Magazine*. He has been featured in the *Wall Street Journal*, the *New York Times*, *Outside Magazine*, *Men's Fitness*, and *Men's Health*. Contact Matt through his website, purplepatchfitness.com.

Matt lives in San Francisco with his wife, Kelli, their son, Baxter, and naughty dog, Willow.